Heart Failure

Heart Failure

A CLINICAL NURSING HANDBOOK

CHRISTOPHER NICHOLSON
BA (Hons), MSc (Clinical Nursing), RGN
Cardiac Nurse Specialist – Heart Failure
Central Lancashire PCT

John Wiley & Sons, Ltd

Other Wiley Editorial Offices

John Wiley & Sons Inc., 111 River Street, Hoboken, NJ 07030, USA

Jossey-Bass, 989 Market Street, San Francisco, CA 94103-1741, USA

Wiley-VCH Verlag GmbH, Boschstr. 12, D-69469 Weinheim, Germany

John Wiley & Sons Australia Ltd, 42 McDougall Street, Milton, Queensland 4064, Australia

John Wiley & Sons (Asia) Pte Ltd, 2 Clementi Loop #02-01, Jin Xing Distripark, Singapore 129809

John Wiley & Sons Canada Ltd, 6045 Freemont Blvd, Mississauga, ONT, L5R 4J3, Canada

Wiley also publishes its books in a variety of electronic formats. Some content that appears in print
may not be available in electronic books.

Anniversary Logo Design: Richard J. Pacifico

Library of Congress Cataloging-in-Publication Data

Nicholson, Christopher, RGN.
  Heart failure : a clinical nursing handbook / Christopher Nicholson.
     p. ; cm.
  Includes bibliographical references and index.
  ISBN 978-0-470-05760-5 (pbk. : alk. paper)
  1. Congestive heart failure—Nursing—Handbooks, manuals, etc.   I. Title.
  [DNLM: 1. Heart Failure, Congestive—nursing—Great Britain. WY 152.5 N624h 2007]
  RC685.C53N53 2007
  616.1'290231—dc22

                                                                        2007015900

A catalogue record for this book is available from the British Library

ISBN: 978-0-470-05760-5

Typeset in 10/12pt Times by Integra Software Services Pvt. Ltd, Pondicherry, India
Printed and bound in Great Britain by TJ International, Padstow
This book is printed on acid-free paper responsibly manufactured from sustainable forestry
in which at least two trees are planted for each one used for paper production.

Contents

About the Author

Chris Nicholson works as a Heart Failure Specialist Nurse for Central Lancashire PCT where he set up and runs the service. It is a nurse-led, community-based service, with hospital in-reach. The caseload is currently around 350 heart failure patients and the area is a mixed population. Prior to his current job Chris has worked as a nurse and charge nurse on coronary care units in secondary and tertiary cardiac centres and as a Nurse Clinician in Cardiology after having completed his Clinical Masters Degree.

Preface

Susan is a 76-year-old widow with two daughters and five grandchildren. She has been admitted to hospital twice recently with breathlessness. After tests she was told she had heart failure and when her breathing improved a little she was sent home with a bag of new tablets. She does not really understand what the tablets are for; she feels tired all the time and she has not been out of her house because she is frightened her heart is about to stop...

There over a million people with heart failure in the United Kingdom and all nurses have cared for, or will care for, patients like Susan: practice nurses, district nurses and community matrons; hospital nurses working in Accident and Emergency, Medical Assessment Units, Coronary Care Units and medical or elderly care wards; as well as specialist heart failure nurses. The care for patients with heart failure has developed rapidly over the past 20 years. The importance of nurses in maintaining and improving the lives and outcomes for patients with heart failure is recognised in the increased responsibilities they have taken on and the central role they have in providing heart failure services.

Caring for patients with heart failure is challenging. It is a complex syndrome. Patients with heart failure have a worse prognosis than almost all forms of cancer, are at risk of acute exacerbations and often live with debilitating symptoms. Some patients with heart failure might perhaps have fewer physical problems but may be suffering from psychological distress because of their condition.

This book is written as a handbook for both practising nurses and students. It provides information on all the major areas of heart failure nursing from diagnosis through to end-stage heart failure. It is designed to be both a quick reference book for the busy practitioner needing to check a clinical question and as a source for wider discussion and analysis of heart failure issues. The book provides key references and highlights areas where the evidence is weak or where there are controversies and disagreements.

It is written with the nurse in mind but would be of use to any professional who cares for patients with heart failure as part of their role, such as physiotherapists and occupational therapists.

Heart failure is a universal healthcare issue but there are differences in care and service provision across the world. This book is based on heart failure care in the United Kingdom but international comparisons and examples are given where helpful.

The book is divided into four parts. The first part is background information and discussions: this is divided into chapters that look at definitions, epidemiology, causes, outcomes and physiology. The second part looks at assessing people with heart failure, for diagnosis and review, with chapters exploring clinical assessment and investigations. The third part considers treatment from education and information, through exercise, medications, surgery and pacemaker devices, up to care of the patient with end-stage heart failure. The fourth part considers policy and service issues, with a chapter explaining the public policy framework within which heart failure services are provided and a chapter looking in detail at issues of setting up and running heart failure services. The final part of the book is for reference, with a list of key heart failure clinical trials, a glossary, references and an index.

Part I   Introduction

1 Definitions

In this chapter heart failure is introduced and a brief historical outline of the condition is given before moving on to explain the terminology and classifications used to describe and define heart failure. There are discussions of the confusion of language, the impact on patients and the effects of definition on healthcare service provision.

INTRODUCTION

Heart failure is a powerful but imprecise phrase. If you asked a dozen patients or clinicians to define heart failure then you would get at least a dozen different answers. One common theme would be that heart failure is serious. Everyone understands that the heart is essential for life, so to hear it is 'failing' is, at the very least, worrying for patients and their carers. The phrase is imprecise because it does not explain if the heart is failing completely or partially, imminently or in the future, permanently or temporarily, what the cause is and whether a cure is possible.

Patients are often unsure what heart failure means for them. Sometimes they think that heart failure is a disease. It is not; it is a syndrome – a collection of signs and symptoms indicating certain anatomical and physiological changes. Heart failure is the end result of a number of diseases – for example, ischaemic heart disease – but is not in itself a disease. For many patients the phrase heart failure might be understood to mean the heart is about to stop. Heart failure does increase the risk of sudden death but that is not what heart failure means: the phrase is a clinical diagnosis – meaning a syndrome characterised by a reduction in the heart's pumping function, with associated complications.

Many eminent clinicians and scholars have attempted to define heart failure more precisely (see Box 1.2). This can be done in a number of ways: for example, it can be described in terms of the structural changes in the heart muscle; or the functional changes in how the heart performs; or it can be described as either acute or chronic depending on its presentation. Whilst in some ways helpful these definitions can also hinder understanding – a patient with structural changes will also have functional changes sooner or later and a patient with acute heart failure only rarely does not also have a background of chronic heart failure, even if undiagnosed.

Box 1.1 A Basic, Functional Definition of Heart Failure

- Heart failure is the failure of the heart to supply (by a pumping action) the volume of blood required to match the demands of the body.
- This reduction in supply is due to a number of potential causes but usually is the failure of the left ventricle to contract well enough.
- The mismatch between supply and demand occurs when demand is at its highest – i.e. on exertion – however, if supply is very poor then it can occur when demand is still relatively low – i.e. at rest.

HISTORICAL OUTLINE

Discussions of heart failure rightly concentrate on current discoveries and treatments so it is sometimes forgotten that heart failure is not a new condition and that understanding of the condition has come about incrementally. An appreciation of the history of the condition is a reminder that current understanding will also be incomplete and perhaps even simply wrong in some respects – a useful point to bear in mind when patients respond differently to expectations.

There are descriptions in classical literature that fit the clinical picture of heart failure (Davis et al. 2000). The Romans were aware of the medicinal (and toxic) effects of the foxglove (digitalis) plant on the heart. This knowledge was passed on through folklore before rediscovery by the medical profession in 1785 by William Withering, a Birmingham physician, who published a paper on digitalis, having seen a woman use it for a patient suffering with *dropsy* – what we would describe as congestive cardiac failure (Bessen 1986).

From the nineteenth century through to the twentieth century the development of investigations such as X-rays, electrocardiographs, echocardiographs and cardiac catheterisations has helped our understanding of what happens when the heart fails. These developments continue with the use of magnetic resonance imaging (MRI) and computer modelling techniques.

Effective treatments have taken longer to emerge. In medieval and early modern times patients with heart failure had, like the sufferers of most conditions, blood drained. This was based on the classical belief that the body had four humours and that an excess of blood caused certain conditions (Ventura & Mehra 2005). It is difficult to imagine that this did anything but make the situation worse physiologically by leading to anaemia and a compensatory neurohormonal response. However, it was the expected treatment of the time and no doubt it had a positive placebo effect for some patients. In the nineteenth and twentieth centuries a slightly different treatment emerged – that of fluid removal from oedematous tissue by inserting drainage tubes, invented by Dr Southey and hence known as Southey Tubes, into the subcutaneous tissues (Davis et al 2000). This may have provided some local improvements in the oedema but it was not treating the cause of the oedema and any improvement would have been only temporary.

Fluid removal continues to be a mainstay of treatment in heart failure patients with fluid retention but it is now removed chemically by drugs rather than mechanically. Diuretics, or drugs that make urine production increase, came into wide clinical practice in the 1950s and remove excess fluid from the body. In the late twentieth century a better understanding of the neurohormonal responses in heart failure led to the development and use of drug therapies to affect these: angiotensin-converting-enzyme inhibitors, angiotensin II receptor blockers and aldosterone antagonists for the renin-angiotensin-aldosterone system; beta-blockers for the adrenergic system.

From the late twentieth century surgical and technological treatments have been developed for patients with heart failure. These include pacemakers, internal defibrillators and surgical treatments. For some patients there are the options of replacing the heart through a transplant or an artificial cardiac support device.

Although heart failure has no doubt been around for as long as humans have existed, it has become a more prominent condition in recent years. This is partly due to advances made in recognition and diagnosis but mainly it is due to the fact that as people live longer it becomes more common. This is for two reasons: firstly, older people are more likely to have had primary cardiac events that may damage their hearts and have had longer exposure to cardiac risk factors; and secondly, the heart, like all organs, naturally loses efficiency and robustness as it ages.

DEFINITIONS

Patients are, not surprisingly, keen to have their condition defined – to get an answer to the simple question, *'What is heart failure'?* Unfortunately for clinicians it is not an easy question to answer simply. Eminent cardiologists have come up with different definitions (see Box 1.2).

Box 1.2 Expert Definitions of Heart Failure

'A condition in which the heart fails to discharge its contents adequately.'
(Lewis 1933)

'A pathophysiological state in which an abnormality of cardiac function is responsible for the failure of the heart to pump blood at a rate commensurate with the requirements of the metabolising tissues.'
(Braunwald 1980)

'A clinical syndrome caused by an abnormality of the heart and recognised by a characteristic pattern of haemodynamic, renal, neural and hormonal responses.'
(Poole-Wilson 1985)

Box 1.2 (Continued)

'Symptoms of heart failure, objective evidence of cardiac dysfunction and response to treatment directed towards heart failure.'

(Task Force of the European Society of Cardiology 1995)

'Heart Failure is a complex syndrome that can result from any structural or functional cardiac disorder that impairs the ability of the heart to function as a pump to support a physiological circulation. The syndrome of heart failure is characterised by symptoms such as breathlessness and fatigue, and signs such as fluid retention.'

(National Institute for Clinical Excellence 2003)

Quotations from Davis et al. 2000 and NICE 2003

There are various problems with defining heart failure for patients and heart failure is an uncomfortable diagnosis for patients, clinicians and health service managers.

For patients the phrase is highly value-laden. Patients know that anything to do with the heart is serious and potentially fatal. The word 'failure' has a socially constructed meaning that is negative: it is the opposite of success. There is also, for some, an implication that the individual has responsibility for the failure. We all want to be successful and are often regaled with anecdotes about how our successes or failures are up to ourselves. A parallel might be drawn with cancer patients and the way in which patients can feel under societal pressure to 'stay positive'. It is curious how this pressure seems to apply only to conditions that are either life-threatening or have limited treatments: there does not seem to be a parallel pressure to stay positive, as a determinate of the success of the treatment, when having a cataract operation.

As noted earlier, for patients the phrase is unclear – does it mean that the heart is about to stop? Patients also easily confuse heart failure, myocardial infarction and arrhythmia. This is hardly surprising as they are linked and patients could of course have them simultaneously. Psychologically, the phrase heart failure and the explanation that it is a progressive and chronic condition are difficult for the patient to deal with as people are used to stories of medical interventions and successes and expect something to be available as a cure. It is important that definitions are clear and comprehensible. This means clinicians must avoid jargon, medicalisation and over-complication. It means clinicians must be ready to adapt their explanations to suit the patient's understanding. Communication failures are, regrettably, quite common in clinical practice – for example, in one study of heart failure 40 % of patients had no understanding of the nature or seriousness of their condition (Buetow & Coster 2001b). It is sensible practice to check patients' understanding in later consultations and to build up their knowledge gradually – see Chapter 8.

For the clinician the problem with the phrase heart failure is that it is so broad. Although heart failure is usually a functional phrase it is imprecise: a heart may be failing in the sense that it is not going to last another 24 hours; or it may be failing in the sense that a weakness has been diagnosed for many years; or even, taking the American Heart Association staging system, that there are risk factors or precipitating diseases for heart failure. It is also imprecise as a definition because the heart can fail in different ways – hence the use of more structural terms such as left-sided, right-sided, biventricular and congestive cardiac failure. It is also possible to define heart failure using descriptive terms such as high output, low output, diastolic and systolic dysfunction. Other definitions try to link to specific changes in the structure or tissues of the heart muscle – such as dilated cardiomyopathy – sometimes with the addition of the underlying cause – such as alcoholic dilated cardiomyopathy. The common criticism of these definitions is that they are reductionist. It could also be argued that defining conditions in medical terminology eases the explanation process for the clinician by medicalising the condition but excludes the patients by setting up a professional terminology barrier. The risk of telling the patient that they have *dilated cardiomyopathy* is that they might have no idea that it means they have *heart failure*. Various clinicians have advanced alternative phrases to heart failure but even the relatively minor adjustment from *heart failure* to *cardiac failure* is a move away from plain English.

For the health service the problem of the definition of heart failure is also a real one. This is because in order to tackle, analyse and resource a problem you need to know what the problem is and what it is not, how widespread it is and what resources it uses. Using a closed definition of heart failure (such as left ventricular systolic dysfunction confirmed on echocardiogram, as in the new GP contracts), a smaller number of patients will be found than if a broader definition (such as including diastolic dysfunction and those with clinical evidence but no echocardiogram confirmation) is used. Using a broader definition of heart failure may be best if the policy aim is to reduce the burden of heart failure or future presentation. Conversely, if the aim is to target resources to those with existing symptomatic heart failure, a narrower definition of heart failure is best. For health service managers a further complication with definitions is that different types of heart failure need different types of funding – a patient with genetic cardiomyopathy may not have many admissions but if they do they may be high cost; and as they are diagnosed younger than the average heart failure patient, their healthcare costs are over many more years.

TERMINOLOGY

CARDIOMYOPATHY

The term cardiomyopathy began being used in the 1950s and was first classified by the World Health Organization in 1980 (World Health Organization 1980).

Cardiomyopathy means disease of the heart muscle. The World Health Organization definition can cover the majority of cases of heart failure, the exceptions being reversible functional causes such as acute anaemia and thyrotoxicosis.

Box 1.3 WHO Cardiomyopathy Classification

Intrinsic to myocardium

- Dilated Cardiomyopathy (DCM)
- Hypertrophic Cardiomyopathy (HCM)
- Arrythromogenic Right Ventricular Dysplasia (ARVD)
- Obliterative Cardiomyopathy (OCM)

Secondary to external processes

- Ischaemic Cardiomyopathy
- Hypertensive Cardiomyopathy
- Valvular Cardiomyopathy
- Inflammatory Cardiomyopathy
- Cardiomyopathy due to other systemic diseases.

A more detailed classification of cardiomyopathy is provided by the American Heart Association and has recently been revised (Maron et al. 2006).

Box 1.4 AHA/ACC Cardiomyopathy Classification

Primary Cardiomyopathies

Genetic	• Hypertrophic Cardiomyopathy • Arrythmogenic Right Ventricular Dysplasia (ARVD) • Conduction System Disease (Lenerge Disease) • Ion Channel Diseases (Long QT Syndrome; Brugada Syndrome; Catecholaminergic Polymorphic Ventricular Tachycardia; Short QT Syndrome; Idiopathic Ventricular Fibrillation)
Mixed (Genetic and Non-genetic)	• Dilated Cardiomyopathy • Primary Restrictive Non-hypertrophied Cardiomyopathy
Acquired	• Myocarditis (Inflammatory Cardiomyopathy) • Stress ('Tako-Tsubo') Cardiomyopathy • Peripartum Cardiomyopathy • Arrhythmia Induced Cardiomyopathy • Alcoholic Cardiomyopathy

---

Box 1.4 (Continued)

Secondary Cardiomyopathy

Infiltrative	• Amyloidosis • Gaucher Disease • Hurler's Disease • Hunter's Disease
Storage	• Haemochromatosis • Fabry's Disease • Glycogen Storage Disease • Niemann-Pick Disease
Toxicity	• Drugs • Heavy Metals • Chemicals
Endomyocardial	• Endomyocardial Fibrosis • Loeffler's Endocarditis
Inflammatory	• Sarcoidosis
Endocrine	• Diabetes Mellitus • Hyperthyroidism • Hypothyroidism • Hyperparathyroidism • Phaeochromocytoma • Acromegaly
Cardiofacial	• Noonan Syndrome • Lentiginosis
Neuromuscular/Neurological	• Friedriech's Ataxia • Duchenne-Becker Muscular Dystrophy • Myotonic Dystrophy • Tuberous Sclerosis
Nutritional Deficiencies	• Beriberi (Thiamine Deficiency) • Pallagra • Scurvy • Selenium • Carnitine • Kwashiorkor
Autoimmune/Collagen	• Systemic Lupus Erythema • Dermatomyositis • Rheumatoid Arthritis • Scleroderma • Polyarteritis Nodosa • Electrolyte Imbalance
Post-cancer treatment	• Radiation • Anthracyclines • Cyclophosphamide

As can be seen from these classification systems the term cardiomyopathy can be helpful when trying to move from a clinical diagnosis based on presentation and investigation to consideration of the underlying cause of the condition. It is important to try to do this because, as the lists clearly show, there are a great many potential causes of cardiomyopathy and they have different implications for patients and their families. However, in clinical practice, patients often present with several possible causes of heart failure and it is not always possible to determine where they would fit in a classification system.

LEFT VENTRICULAR FAILURE (LVF)

Left ventricular failure is often the admission diagnosis of acutely unwell patients admitted to hospital with heart failure. Left ventricular failure is also the usual cause of chronic symptoms such as breathlessness in patients with heart failure.

The left ventricle is the heart chamber that pumps blood through the aortic valve into circulation. In order to do so it has the highest pressure and largest muscle bulk of any of the heart chambers. There are several ways in which the left ventricle can fail. It may fail either acutely or chronically. It can be too baggy (dilated), or the chamber size might be too small because the muscle is over-thickened (hypertrophy). There might be problems with the ability of the muscle to contract – either the power or the co-ordination of the contractions.

The most common left ventricular problem in developed countries is as a consequence (either immediate or longer term) of ischaemic heart disease. The workload of the left ventricle creates a high demand for blood. The left ventricle has the largest coronary blood supply, making it the most likely to be involved in myocardial infarctions. Damage to the left ventricular myocardium through infarction leads to reduced contractility and abnormal movement of the walls. The result is either reduced cardiac output or a need for the ventricle to increase its workload to maintain the same cardiac output. This in turn leads to an increase in muscle bulk (hypertrophy) and an enlargement of the chamber (dilation).

These physical changes in the myocardium are known as remodelling and are mediated by the effects of hormones. Although a compensatory mechanism the remodelling of the heart has a negative effect eventually as the ventricle, in effect, becomes 'over-stretched' and the fibres lose their elasticity. This is discussed more in Chapter 5.

RIGHT VENTRICULAR FAILURE (RVF)

Although the left ventricle is the most common ventricle to fail (and some people mistakenly assume left ventricular failure and heart failure are synonymous) it is possible that the right ventricle can fail without the initial involvement of the left ventricle.

This can occur in right ventricular myocardial infarctions or in patients who have severe lung disease. Patients who develop right-sided heart failure as a secondary result of lung disease are said to have *cor pulmonale.*

Right ventricular failure presents differently to left ventricular failure and this will be discussed in Chapter 6. Eventually, a failing right ventricle will lead to a failing left ventricle just as a failing left ventricle eventually leads to a failing right ventricle.

BIVENTRICULAR FAILURE OR CONGESTIVE CARDIAC FAILURE (CCF)

This is the term used when both ventricles are failing simultaneously. As you would expect, biventricular failure is suggestive of a more advanced heart failure, with more complications and worse outcomes. The term congestive cardiac failure was used in order to describe the pattern of fluid retention and pulmonary oedema usually present. It is a phrase which has fallen out of favour recently because congestion is not always present (particularly if the patient is managed well) and biventricular failure is the preferred phrase.

LEFT VENTRICULAR SYSTOLIC DYSFUNCTION (LVSD)

At present the term 'left ventricular systolic dysfunction' is often used, incorrectly, as a surrogate for heart failure. It describes the left ventricle not contracting properly and could be considered a sub-division of left ventricular failure. It is the most common form of heart failure in the developed world because it is the usual pattern of heart failure after myocardial infarction. It is characterised on echocardiogram by non-contracting (akinetic) or poorly contracting (hypokinetic) areas of the left ventricular wall.

The reason why left ventricular systolic dysfunction is widely used as a definition of heart failure is because it is easy to detect on echocardiogram. This makes it a simple marker to look for in trials or as part of screening programmes or registers. For these reasons, confirming left ventricular systolic dysfunction on echocardiogram is used as one of the quality markers in the GMS contract, the system by which GPs are rewarded for meeting health targets in the UK. The problem with using left ventricular systolic function in this way is that it ignores heart failure with preserved left ventricular function – a significant group that includes around 40 % of the whole heart failure population.

DIASTOLIC HEART FAILURE

Until relatively recently diastolic heart failure was a controversial definition. This was because it is difficult to find objective evidence for diastolic dysfunction with the diagnostic tests we have. Diastolic dysfunction occurs when the heart does not relax properly after systole. This may be caused by scarring, hypertension or the fibrotic changes of old age. It is thought that diastolic heart failure may account for the clinically observed fact that some patients seem to have all the signs and symptoms of heart failure but have preserved left ventricular systolic function on echocardiogram (Andrew 2003). It is estimated that 40% of patients with heart failure may have diastolic dysfunction. In the CHARMES study diastolic dysfunction was found on the echocardiogram of two thirds of patients hospitalised with symptoms of heart failure but who had preserved systolic function (Persson et al. 2007).

LEFT VENTRICULAR HYPERTROPHY (LVH)

Although left ventricular hypertrophy is not strictly speaking a term that describes heart failure it is worth considering because of its close physiological links. It describes an increase in the muscle mass of the left ventricle. This is usually caused as a response to either myocardial infarction or chronic hypertension. As a result of these causes, the discovery of left ventricular hypertrophy on an electrocardiogram or echocardiogram is an important finding. Even if no overt heart failure is found the patient is at high risk of developing heart failure in the future and should be treated and followed up closely.

GRADING OF HEART FAILURE

We have seen that there are many definitions available for heart failure. There are also several ways that heart failure can be graded. As well as the structural and descriptive classification discussed earlier it is possible to attempt to grade severity by objective measurements.

One way to do this is to calculate the left ventricular ejection fraction (LVEF) – the percentage of blood that leaves the left ventricle into circulation. As the usual stroke volume is around 70 ml and the typical left ventricular end-diastolic volume 120 ml, the ejection fraction is 70 divided by 120, which is 0.6 or 60%. The ejection fraction is a way of quantifying left ventricular systolic dysfunction. The rationale for being interested in the ejection fraction is that the worse the ejection fraction the more severe the potential heart failure. This has some validity, although it needs to be stressed that individual patients with a poor ejection fraction may be asymptomatic, or a particular patient with a good ejection fraction may have severe symptoms. The degree of reduction of left ventricular ejection fraction is often measured as part of the demographics and inclusion/exclusion criteria of clinical trials in heart failure.

Box 1.5 Left Ventricle Ejection Fraction and Systolic Dysfunction

LVEF%	Systolic Dysfunction
60%	Normal
45–60%	Mild left ventricular dysfunction
35–45%	Moderate left ventricular dysfunction
25–35%	Severe left ventricular dysfunction
< 25%	Extremely severe left ventricular dysfunction

A widely used method for classifying heart failure is the New York Heart Association (NYHA) grading. This has been in use since 1928 and provides a four-stage classification based on the patient's symptoms (Subramanian et al. 2005). It has the advantages of being both easy to remember and a simple practical method for testing whether someone has improved or worsened. It is not, however, infallible as some observer bias is inevitable and it relies on patient self-reported information. It is also limited in that it is difficult to assess the NYHA grade in patients with respiratory conditions.

Box 1.6 New York Heart Association (NYHA) Classification

Class I: Asymptomatic
Class II: Symptoms on maximal exertion
Class III: Symptoms on minimal exertion
Class IV: Symptoms at rest

In 1998 the American Heart Association and the American College of Cardiology introduced a classification scheme to stage heart failure. This is based on the successful staging system used in cancer care. The purpose is to recognise that heart failure is a continuum and to refocus attention on patients who are at risk of heart failure or in the early stages, so that they receive treatment long before they become acutely unwell.

Box 1.7 AHA/ACC Heart Failure Staging Classification

A No clinical, structural or functional signs of heart failure but at high risk of developing heart failure due to co-morbidities (such as hypertension, ischaemic heart disease, alcoholism, rheumatic fever, etc.)

Box 1.7 (Continued)

B No clinical signs or symptoms of heart failure but evidence of structural heart disease (such as left ventricular dilation or hypertrophy, previous myocardial infarction or valve disease)
C Symptoms of heart failure and underlying structural heart disease
D Symptoms of heart failure at rest, despite treatment optimisation, with advanced structural heart disease

(Hunt et al. 2001)

2 Epidemiology

In this chapter the epidemiological data for heart failure are outlined. The emphasis is on United Kingdom data but international comparisons are also drawn. The data are interpreted to make sense at different levels: from the national context, to the local hospital and general practice levels. Studies and reports making predictions for the future heart failure population are also noted and the effect this may have on service provision considered.

OVERVIEW

In order to understand the problem of heart failure it is important to study its scope – how many people have it (*prevalence*) and how many new cases there are every year in the population (*incidence*). It is also important to consider these issues for different groups and localities within the overall population in case there are differences within subgroups. Are there gender, racial or geographical differences that will lead to different levels or types of health needs? Having epidemiological baselines allows comparisons of one area against another, reducing the likelihood of making assumptions that are not true reflections of local circumstances and enabling better planning and delivery of services.

We have seen in the preceding chapter that it is very difficult to come up with a precise definition of heart failure that covers all the differences within the condition. Not surprisingly, therefore, when people have looked at how often heart failure occurs and with what frequency in different populations at different times, there have been very different answers. No doubt this is mainly due to the imprecision of the definition but another factor is that studies tend to find what they look for. For example, if you record all myocardial infarctions and follow these patients closely for a long time then more heart failure will be found, as myocardial infarction by definition causes muscle damage, which will lead to future inefficiency even if not evident immediately. So, at which point would you say that the patient having had a myocardial infarction has heart failure – when the echocardiogram shows systolic dysfunction, or when there are clinical signs or symptoms of heart failure, or both? Similarly, if you recognise hypertension as a precedent to heart failure and then follow up all hypertensive patients, you will find more heart failure. The increased awareness of heart failure being recognised as a syndrome means it is medicalised and recorded whereas once end stage heart failure might not have been so labelled – being seen as an inevitable precursor to death in the aged. As we discover more precipitating causes for heart failure it may be that the rates of heart failure overall will also increase.

When considering the scope of heart failure, there are several problems that complicate the issue. Firstly, as we have just noted, there is the problem of defining heart failure. We have already seen in Chapter 1 that if we apply a tight definition, such as echocardiogram evidence of left ventricular systolic dysfunction, then we hone in on a much smaller population than if we used a broader definition, based on, say, signs and symptoms of heart failure. The second problem is applying the definition – what is the data source? There is no national population database of medical histories that could simply be searched for heart failure (although this may well become the case if the current policy to hold a national computerised clinical record for every NHS patient is successfully implemented). There are currently extensive local records – at hospitals and GP surgeries – but these are fragmentary and not linked. There is also an issue of data quality within those records with particular concern around coding.

When patients are admitted to hospital information is coded to enable the episode of care to be logged and resources planned. In principle these data should list all heart failure episodes of care. There are several concerns over the accuracy of this coded information. There are several available codes for heart failure – due to historical reasons and the definition difficulties discussed earlier – and this can lead to confusion and missed data. Coding tends to take place based on initial diagnosis and is rarely altered on the basis of final diagnosis. This is an important reason for the misreporting of heart failure because an initial assessment of shortness of breath or difficulty in breathing may be considered heart failure but may later be diagnosed differently. A final point about hospital coding is that it reduces a possibly complex episode to a bare entry and some data richness is lost. For example, a patient in heart failure who is admitted due to a chest infection may have had chronic heart failure for a while without being symptomatic or diagnosed. The physiological stress of the infection may have changed their heart failure from chronic to acute, leading to its discovery. In this case the coding may be chest infection but the patient may well not have required admission if they had not also had heart failure.

Various other methods help to build our knowledge of the extent of heart failure. One method is to look for registries of known patients. With the new GMS contract GP practices have been rewarded for keeping a register of all patients with left ventricular dysfunction. Clinical trials concerned with heart failure contain a designated sample or registry. Longitudinal and cohort studies often take large samples of heart failure populations over a specific geographical location. All of these are samples of varying degrees of usefulness but it must be remembered that they do not sample the entire population and their representativeness must not be taken for granted. An illustration of this point would be clinical trials, from which the elderly are often excluded.

Box 2.1 Epidemiological Studies of Heart Failure

Framingham Heart Study

This famous American longitudinal cohort study started in 1948 with 5209 subjects who were assessed biennially for cardiovascular risk, disease and outcomes. A further cohort of their offspring was added in 1971.

Hillingdon Heart Study

A study over a whole PCT (primary care trust) area in West London, covering 82 general practices, during 1995–96, looking specifically at heart failure epidemiology.

MONICA

Heart failure prevalence study in north Glasgow of 1640 randomly selected patients defining heart failure on clinical grounds and a left ventricular ejection fraction of < 30 %.

ECHOES

Echocardiographic Heart of England Screening study took place in the West Midlands. It defined heart failure on clinical grounds and if left ventricular ejection fraction was < 40 %. A Primary Care-based study of 6286 patients randomly selected in 16 general practices in 1995–99.

Nottingham

This study calculated heart failure prevalence by looking at the prescription of frusemide across Nottingham in 1991–92 and compared with GP notes in 903 patients, finding 56 % of those on frusemide had heart failure.

PREVALENCE

The proportion of people in an entire population who have heart failure at that point in time is the prevalence of heart failure. The people included may have had heart failure for six days or six years – the prevalence figure is only a snapshot for that moment in time.

The NICE guidelines quote heart failure prevalence figures for the United Kingdom of 3–20 per 1000 (0.3 % to 2 %) rising to 30–130 per 1000 (3–13 %)

in the over 75s (NICE 2003). This can be extrapolated to a United Kingdom heart failure population of almost 1 million patients. Another way to express this is to think of an average GP with 2000 patients having around 20–30 patients with heart failure. These NICE figures derive from a range of studies and it is clear that there is considerable variation in these estimates.

Box 2.2 Heart Failure Prevalence Data

Study	Lowest Calculation	Highest Calculation
Hillingdon	9 in 1000 (0.9 %)	74 in 1000 (7.4 %)
Nottingham	1 in 1000 (0.1 %)	55 in 1000 (5.5 %)
MONICA	12 in 1000 (1.2 %)	29 in 1000 (2.9 %)
ECHOES	18 in 1000 (1.8 %)	31 in 1000 (3.1 %)
Framingham	8 in 1000 (0.8 %)	79 in 1000 (7.9 %)

The Hillingdon study looked at data based on the diagnosis of heart failure following hospital admission or attendance at a rapid access clinic (Cowie et al. 1999). In the Nottingham study the prevalence of heart failure was estimated from GP notes (an initial screen was made for patients prescribed loop diuretics) (Clarke et al. 1995). This is probably an underestimation as patients with mild and asymptomatic heart failure may well be excluded as they would be less likely to be prescribed diuretics. Two surveys in the 1990s, in Glasgow (McDonagh et al. 1997) and the West Midlands (Davies et al. 2001), reported left ventricular systolic dysfunction prevalence in 25–74-year-olds and over 45s, respectively. As urban Scotland is known to have very high rates of ischaemic heart disease it may be that the differences between these two surveys regarding prevalence rates is a real one rather than methodological. Clearly, including only patients with evidence of left ventricular systolic dysfunction means that some patients with heart failure – those without an echocardiogram and those with diastolic dysfunction – would be excluded and so the figures may be an underestimation of the true prevalence.

It is interesting to compare the figures from the Framingham study in the United States, which looked at prevalence in people in their 40s to 80s (Kannel and Belanger 1991; Kannel 2000). These figures are in the middle of the range of the results from the United Kingdom-based studies. In the Rotterdam study the prevalence figure was 3.9 % (Mosterd et al. 1999).

The wide variation in prevalence figures within the studies is no doubt due to a combination of different research techniques and real differences in prevalence within the study populations due to socio-economic and medical variations. It is also important when considering the numbers to think about which populations they are from – Framingham is a small town outside Boston in the United States, whereas Hillingdon is an inner London borough – these are not populations from non-Western or undeveloped countries. Common to all of these studies are two features: that prevalence of heart failure rises with age, and that overall prevalence is rising over time.

INCIDENCE

The number of new cases of heart failure, usually given over a year, is the incidence. The reason incidence is a useful number to consider is that it is a measure of risk in a population. Therefore it is useful to services and purchasers for policy and planning.

In the NICE guidelines the incidence of heart failure is given as 1–5 per 1000 per year (0.1 % to 0.5 %) rising to 30 per 1000 per year (3 %) in the over 75s. An average GP with 2000 patients is likely to see around nine patients with suspected heart failure per year and will confirm the diagnosis in three of those patients.

Box 2.3 Heart Failure Incidence Data		
Study	Lowest calculation	Highest calculation
Hillingdon	2 per 10 000 (0.02 %)	12 per 1000 (1.2 %)
Framingham	2 per 1000 (0.2 %)	27 per 1000 (2.7 %)

In the Hillingdon study the overall incidence of heart failure was 0.08 %, from 0.02 % in 45–55-year-olds to 1.2 % in those over 86 years old (Cowie et al. 1999). In this study 80 % of diagnoses were made after an acute hospital admission which might suggest that more acutely unwell patients are being found than patients with chronic heart failure.

In the Framingham study the incidence of heart failure was 0.2 % (2 per 1000) in the age group 45–54, rising to 4 % (40 per 1000) in the group aged 85–94 years. The incidence roughly doubled every decade and the incidence in women was slightly less than for men at all ages (Kannel and Belanger 1991). A problem with the Framingham Study is that the diagnosis of heart failure was made on clinical grounds and there was no routine confirmation of dysfunction using an echocardiogram. This was standard practice when the study started but it does mean that the epidemiological data may not be fully accurate.

SUBGROUP DIFFERENCES

While the overall prevalence and incidence figures are important for healthcare planning, they are broad figures that can mask important variations within different subgroups of the population.

ASYMPTOMATIC PATIENTS

Most of the epidemiological studies rely on the patient having signs or symptoms of heart failure at the very least, often also requiring a degree of confirmation by echocardiographic evidence. However, not all patients with heart failure have symptoms – a fact that is recognised in the NYHA classifications grade I. None of the studies have taken an entire population and screened them all for heart failure. If this approach was taken then the asymptomatic patients would also be included. This would increase prevalence and incidence rates substantially. Screening programmes could also be carried out to look for patients with predisposing conditions placing them at the early stages of heart failure. The counter arguments against screening programmes are: firstly, that we do not necessarily understand enough about the natural history of heart failure for very early detection to be necessarily useful; secondly, it would be extremely expensive; and thirdly, a lot of patients would be labelled with the condition.

GENDER

There has been a range of gender differences – in terms of diagnosis, treatment and outcomes – in patients with heart disease (Stramba-Badiale et al. 2006). The incidence of heart failure in most studies is slightly higher for men and this is usually attributed to higher rates of detected ischaemic heart disease. Although women continue to have better life expectancy, the prevalence numbers for heart failure are, however, similar between the sexes. Two United States Medicare databases – the Cooperative Cardiovascular Project and the National Heart Failure Project – did not demonstrate any significant gender bias in the treatment of women with heart failure (Gold & Krumholz 2006).

ELDERLY PATIENTS

Heart failure is a condition of old age in that the median age on presentation is around 75 years old (Cowie et al. 2000). The heart function tends to decline with age like all the organs and the older someone is the more years risk factors and co-morbidities have had to affect the heart. There are of course many younger patients with heart failure too. A consistent pattern within studies is that both prevalence and incidence steadily increase with age, doubling every decade in the Framingham study, for example (Kannel 2000).

RACE

There are very few data on how ethnicity may affect heart failure and most trial populations have been predominately white (Sosin et al. 2004). Studies have found ethnic differences in prevalence: Afro-American men have been reported as being a third more likely to be admitted with heart failure than white men, and black women half as likely again as white women (Menash et al. 2005). A similar pattern was found in a survey in a United States teaching hospital where Afro-Americans were less likely than whites to receive cardiology specialised care if admitted with heart failure (Ahmed et al. 2003a). Ethnic differences in heart failure may be partly due to different underlying causes – hypertension and diabetes being more common in black and subcontinent Asian patients, for example.

FUTURE TRENDS

It is widely agreed that the number of patients with heart failure is likely to rise for the foreseeable future (NICE 2003). This growth in heart failure patients has been due largely to patients living longer and better survival rates for acute cardiac events. It is reasonable to assume these trends will probably continue.

As more community-based screening takes place and as the profile of heart failure rises the number of patients diagnosed, especially those who have mild symptoms or are asymptomatic, is likely to rise. If developments in risk factor analysis or improvements in genetic testing enable patients with a predisposition to heart failure to be recognised before they develop the syndrome, then the numbers will increase. Better technology and interpretation will probably enable diastolic heart failure to be diagnosed with more accuracy and certainty.

The prevalence of patients with heart failure will also be increased by developments in heart failure treatment. Research shows that medications such as ACE-inhibitors, spironolactone and beta-blockers increase survival. Survival has also been improved in clinical trials of regular exercise programmes and of internal cardiac defibrillators. These trials have taken place over the last 20 years and these are now standard treatments. It would be reasonable to assume that over the next 20 years there will also be major developments – perhaps better cardiac support devices, or stem cell therapy or genetic treatments – in heart failure treatment, which will also help patients to live longer.

Within the heart failure population the balance of patients will also change. As more internal cardiac defibrillators are inserted the numbers of patients dying of sudden arrhythmia will decline. This means that more people will survive into old age, when age and other factors will mean they will die of end-stage heart failure.

3 Causes

In this chapter the causes of heart failure will be discussed. The most common causes of heart failure in the developed world – ischaemic heart disease and hypertension – are presented, along with less common causes. The mechanisms by which they are thought to cause heart failure are outlined. The problems associated with finding specific causes for individual patients are noted. Finally, the debates about risk factors for heart failure and current knowledge of genetic cardiomyopathy are discussed.

OVERVIEW

Finding out why a patient has heart failure is important. Patients want to know what has caused their condition – it is human nature to try to understand and rationalise. Clear explanations of what heart failure is and how it has come about are, psychologically, often the first steps for patients in coming to terms with their condition. Sometimes poor explanations or understanding may lead to misapprehension about the causes and this can have an affect on patients' ability to cope. Occasionally, there is not a clear cause for the heart failure, or perhaps there are a couple of potential causes. None the less, wherever possible, it is usually helpful for the patient to be given a simple explanation as to why they have heart failure, along the lines of,

'Your heart is not pumping as well as before because the heart attack you had has led to some damage to the heart muscle.'

Or,

'Your heart is not pumping as well as before because your high blood pressure has put a strain on the heart muscle and changed its shape.'

Or whatever is applicable for that individual patient.

Clinicians need to be careful to avoid language that implies blame. Although the links between obesity, high blood pressure, diabetes and heart failure are now well understood it is usually not helpful, or necessarily true, to say or imply it is the patient's fault they have heart failure. Such an approach often leads to concordance difficulties. It is better to explain how a healthy lifestyle can improve the patient's symptoms and reduce the effects of the heart failure. Occasionally, patients or their partners may also be looking to blame. An example of this is when the GP is blamed for not requesting tests early enough. Again, looking to blame others and focusing on one 'mistake' is a psychological response that is generally maladaptive and patients should be encouraged to reinterpret their situation with the present and future, rather than the past, at the forefront of their mind.

It is important to try and find the cause of the heart failure for clinical reasons. Some causes of heart failure are reversible, such as acute anaemia or thyrotoxicosis, so correct diagnosis and treatment removes the problem. Other causes of heart failure may be improved by specific treatments – valve surgery in some instances of valve-induced heart failure, for example. Some causes of heart failure will lead to a poor outcome if not addressed – such as alcoholic cardiomyopathy patients who continue to drink; or diabetics who continue to be poorly controlled.

Working out the cause of the heart failure is important because the prognosis may differ. For example, a patient with early onset amyloid heart failure has a very poor prognosis, whereas a patient of similar age with hypertrophic obstructive cardiomyopathy may have a good prognosis, especially if action is taken to reduce the risk of sudden death.

When trying to isolate the cause of heart failure it is important to bear in mind that most patients with heart failure will have chronic heart failure, be elderly and have many other medical problems. This means the heart failure is likely to have been present for a while, have worsened gradually and that there may be many potential causes for the heart failure.

Sometimes no clear cause is found for the heart failure. This is unusual and can be a little frustrating for everyone. It illustrates the fact that heart failure is a syndrome not a disease and there are aspects of it that we do not fully understand.

Deciding what the cause of the heart failure is can be complex. The main clues are to be found in the patient's history. Symptoms and examinations may contribute a little and sometimes the investigations can help to suggest which cause is most likely. For example, a patient with symptoms of left ventricular failure, with a history of myocardial infarction, regional akinesia and hypokinesia of the left ventricle on echocardiogram, is a common presentation for heart failure with a background of ischaemic heart disease. Of course, that sort of patient may well also have a history of hypertension or diabetes. If the patient had the myocardial infarction some time ago then there will have been remodelling of the left ventricle and the picture may also include cardiomegaly on chest X-ray and left ventricular dilation on echocardiogram.

As always in clinical practice, most situations are common, some are less common and there are also numerous very rare situations. Whilst not forgetting about the possibility of rare causes and remembering the less common causes, the fact remains that most patients will have a common cause. In heart failure, this means a division such as that set out in Box 3.1.

Box 3.1 Summary of Causes of Heart Failure

Common Causes of Heart Failure

- Ischaemic Heart Disease
- Hypertension

Less Common Causes of Heart Failure

- Alcohol
- Diabetes
- Familial
- Infection
- Valve Disease
- Arrhythmia

Rare Causes of Heart Failure

- Numerous – see AHA/ACC classification in Chapter 1.

ISCHAEMIC HEART DISEASE

In developed countries the most common cause for heart failure is ischaemic heart disease. Studies suggest it accounts for between half and three-quarters of cases (Mair et al. 1996; Zannad et al. 1999). It is thought to be the largest cause of heart failure in the developed world because people are living longer, with wealthier lifestyles, leading to ischaemic heart disease and myocardial infarction, which patients increasingly survive thanks to modern medicine (Stewart et al. 2003a).

When patients have a myocardial infarction the blood supply to an area of the heart muscle is interrupted, usually due to a clot blocking a coronary artery. If the blood supply is not restored rapidly then the cells that are not supplied with blood burst and an area of muscle dies. This dead area of muscle is no longer able to contract and will show up on echocardiograms as not moving (*akinetic*). The muscle surrounding the infarcted area will have a reduced blood supply (*ischaemia*) and will contract poorly (*hypokinesia*) or in an unco-ordinated manner (*dyskinesia*). As most myocardial infarcts affect the left ventricle, that is the usual area of myocardium that is affected. Over time pathological changes will occur as a result of the infarction, with remodelling of the ventricle leading to a larger and less effective heart.

There are other complications that can occur during, or as a result of, myocardial infarction that lead to heart failure: papillary muscles supporting the valve cusps may be torn and valve incompetence develops, a septal defect may be produced, or the patient may develop arrhythmias.

Patients having an acute myocardial infarction may go into acute left ventricular failure at the same time. Sometimes this can mask the myocardial infarction for clinicians and sometimes the converse is the case as it may alert them to the problem. Not all patients presenting with a myocardial infarction will also have acute left ventricular failure and vice versa.

Patients with ischaemic heart disease are also likely to have other conditions and risk factors that, as well as predisposing them towards their ischaemic heart disease, may also cause heart failure. An example would be hypertension. In the Framingham study over 90 % of the patients with heart failure had a history of ischaemic heart disease and/or hypertension (Kannel and Belanger 1991).

As all myocardial infarctions, by definition, cause a permanent impairment to the heart muscle it could be argued that all patients who have had myocardial infarctions have heart failure even if they do not have any overt signs or symptoms. They would certainly fit the American Heart Association/American College of Cardiology staging A and B criteria for heart failure (Hunt et al. 2001). Traditionally patients would only be considered to have heart failure if there is evidence of significant left ventricular systolic dysfunction on echocardiogram after acute myocardial infarction. This is more than just a matter of definition – if these patients are classified as having heart failure they are likely to have more frequent follow-up and be encouraged to achieve more medication and lifestyle adherence. It could be argued that it is a better use of resources to concentrate on patients at the early stage of heart failure as there is more likelihood of interventions having an impact. As a negative counterpoint, if all myocardial infarction patients are told they have a degree of heart failure then there will be a psychological cost to explaining to people that they have a chronic condition, not just an acute episode. Also, it is not known if all, or which, patients who are asymptomatic after myocardial infarction will go on to develop overt heart failure in the future.

Some patients with ischaemic heart disease have ongoing stable pattern angina. They may also have heart failure. It is difficult to know if angina causes heart failure. There may well be some effects on myocardial contraction through persistent ischaemia even if there has not been an infarction (Elhendy et al. 2005).

Patients with ischaemic heart disease may go on to have coronary revascularisation if they have areas of reversible ischaemia. Post surgery, if they are asymptomatic, should they be considered to have heart failure? Surgery certainly can improve left ventricular function in some patients but it is important to remember that the systemic disease process, arteriosclerosis, is still in place and previous myocardial damage still present. Again, using the American Heart Association/American College of Cardiology staging process it is probably right to continue to view these patients as having chronic heart failure and treat accordingly.

HYPERTENSION

High blood pressure is thought to be the second most common cause of heart failure in the developed world and is common in combination with ischaemic heart disease (Meredith and Östergren 2006). In the Framingham study initial cohort it was the most frequently cited cause of heart failure, although it was overtaken by ischaemic heart disease in subsequent cohorts (Kannel 2000). It is possible for severe malignant hypertension to cause acute heart failure but more common is chronic hypertension causing chronic heart failure.

The mechanisms by which hypertension causes heart failure are connected to both gross ventricular shape and myocardial fibre structure. Increased afterload, or the pressure the heart beats against, causes an increase in muscle tension leading to over-stretch. This leads to left ventricular hypertrophy, which can be seen in the ECG of the patient as tall R waves, downward sloping ST segments and T wave inversion in the lateral chest leads. If on assessment a patient has hypertension and ECG evidence of left ventricular hypertrophy, their risk of heart failure increases by a factor of fifteen compared with a patient without these factors in the Framingham study (Kannel and Belanger 1991). Hypertension seems to be closely associated with the development of diastolic dysfunction in particular (Chinnaiyan et al. 2007).

A problem with hypertension is that it is usually silent and unless the problem is found fortuitously, perhaps on occupational medical screening, the patient will be unaware of it. This may mean that they will have hypertension for some years and the longer they have untreated hypertension the more likely cardiac complications are to develop (Williams et al. 2004). When taking a patient history it is necessary to ask not only if they have high blood pressure – they may say no, but in fact have not had it checked for many years, if at all – but it is also important to find out when it was last checked.

Another point worth noting is that patients on treatment for high blood pressure will hopefully have normalised their blood pressure. However, if they had hypertension for many years before that, damage may already be present in the myocardium.

Even patients with apparently normal, untreated blood pressure may still have had hypertension if they are showing signs or symptoms of heart failure. Their blood pressure may have been high without their knowledge but may have fallen with developing pump failure. This is sometimes described as 'burn-out' hypertension.

Patients with known heart failure should have their hypertension controlled. For patients who have high blood pressure but no evidence of heart failure it is probably wise to consider them at high risk of developing heart failure, as category A on the American College of Cardiology/American Heart Association staging guide, with treatment and monitoring to reflect this higher risk.

VALVE DISEASE

In the Hillingdon Study 7 % of patients with heart failure had valve disease as the cause of their heart failure (Cowie et al. 1999). However, as valve disease becomes more common with age it may be that the valve disease and the heart failure are not linked in some patients but coincidental findings. Further complicating matters is the fact that as the heart fails it can distort in shape and pull the valves so that they become regurgitant, thus the valve disease in these cases is a consequence rather than a cause of heart failure.

The purpose of the heart valves is to control the flow of blood through the chambers of the heart, to the lungs and to systemic circulation. Any problem with the valves reduces the efficiency of the flow of the blood through the heart. The heart then attempts to compensate with changes to pressures within the chambers and the result over time is a further worsening in structure and function. Valve disease leads to heart failure because the cardiac output will drop and compensatory mechanisms are activated.

Valves can be diseased in various ways. It is easiest to think of these functionally: they will either become tighter and difficult to open (*stenosis*); or fail to close tightly and so let some blood flow back (*regurgitant* or *incompetent*); or sometimes a combination of both. Various conditions can lead to these problems, such as rheumatic heart disease, age-related stenosis, myocardial infarction and cardiac infection.

Any of the four cardiac valves may be problematic or a number of the valves may have problems at once. The most common problems are mitral regurgitation and aortic stenosis. The consequences of valve disease can be readily appreciated if you think of the blood flow through the heart. If the aortic valve is too tight then pressures within the left ventricle will rise to compensate, eventually leading to left ventricular hypertrophy and reducing the chamber size of the left ventricle. If the aortic valve is incompetent then blood will back flow into the left ventricle and the volume overload will cause left ventricular dilation. Similarly, a stenosed mitral valve will increase left atrial pressures and an incompetent mitral valve will increase left atrial volume and cause dilation. If the pressure in the left atrium rises too much it may be transferred into the lung arterioles, causing pulmonary oedema and breathlessness. Problems with the valves on the right side are often a result of chronic respiratory disease or hepatic problems.

ARRHYTHMIAS

Abnormal heart rhythms are both a cause of heart failure and a consequence of heart failure. If an arrhythmia has caused acute heart failure and is corrected soon enough then chronic heart failure may be avoided. In these circumstances reverting to a normal rate (and/or rhythm) will remove the problem. It may however be that the arrhythmia has unmasked an underlying weakness in the heart that was not apparent up until then. When the arrhythmia is a consequence of chronic heart failure it is often very difficult to restore sinus rhythm as the conducting tissue may be damaged in shape or function.

Acute heart failure can be provoked by the effects of sudden haemodynamic changes due to a paroxysmal arrhythmia – such as atrial fibrillation. This can be seen in both brady- and tachyarrhythmias but is a more common cause of hospitalisation in tachyarrhythmia.

Chronic atrial fibrillation is very common – especially so as people get older – being present in 10 % of the over 75s generally and up to 30 % of patients with chronic heart failure in the Hillingdon Heart study (Cowie et al. 1999). In atrial fibrillation the flow of the blood through the heart is turbulent and the efficiency of the heart decreases. It further decreases if the rate is high as there is less diastolic filling time, and hence less myocardial stretch and forward flow, as regulated by the Frank-Starling effect (Levick 1995). Restoration of sinus rhythm is the ideal but in chronic atrial fibrillation, especially in the elderly, this is often unsuccessful so the strategy then needs to be rate control and anti-coagulation (Kareti et al. 2005). The role of AV node ablation and biventricular pacing in patients with heart failure and atrial fibrillation is as yet unknown (Stevenson & Tedrow 2006).

INFECTION

Heart failure is sometimes caused by infections of the heart. Infections and consequent inflammation of the heart can occur in the inner lining of the heart (*endocarditis),* within the heart muscle (*myocarditis*), or in the outer lining (*pericarditis*). Although not common, acute viral myocarditis is the most likely reason for heart failure in younger patients (Burian et al 2005).

Acute myocarditis is usually viral but non-viral organisms, such as bacteria, can also cause myocarditis and endocarditis. The coxsackie virus group is found in about a third of cases of myocarditis. Some others viruses thought to potentially cause cases of myocarditis are chickenpox, measles, rubella and mumps. Other infective causes of heart failure include rheumatic fever, Chagas disease and HIV (Burian et al. 2005).

Patients with acute myocarditis or endocarditis often become seriously ill very quickly with symptoms such as fever, myalgia, malaise and sometimes chest pain if the pericardium is involved. Patients may develop acute heart failure and arrhythmias. Sometimes the patient is very unwell, but not always so, and sometimes the only evidence of myocarditis in their history is a mild viral infection – or the patient may even be asymptomatic.

If the patient is acutely unwell then inflammatory markers and other samples may help to make the diagnosis. An echocardiogram can help to identify organisms attached to the cardiac valves in the case of endocarditis. Cardiac biopsy is sometimes performed but is rarely helpful in clinical practice. Diagnosis is principally based on the history and sometimes a diagnosis of myocarditis is proposed in cases of heart failure where there is no other obvious cause.

Following the acute episode the patient may recover well although there is a high initial mortality with endocarditis (Hill et al. 2007). Where biopsies have been done the inflammatory changes in the tissues of the muscle fibres and inflammatory cells in the interstitial tissue are permanent, so even if these patients show no signs or symptoms of heart failure it is reasonable to assume they do have heart failure.

ALCOHOL

Patients with a history of alcohol abuse can develop a particular type of heart failure known as alcoholic cardiomyopathy. It is probably a larger cause of heart failure than previously thought but perhaps under-represented in studies as alcoholics are not likely to be included in clinical trials and often are not in regular contact with the health services (Piano & Schwertz 1994; Lee & Regan 2002; Piano 2002).

Alcoholics with heart failure tend to have a globular dilated cardiomyopathy. When they present depends upon their history of alcohol abuse – most commonly it will be in their forties or fifties, usually a little younger than patients with ischaemic cardiomyopathy. A minority of all alcohol drinkers will develop heart failure – there appears to be a genetic predisposition to both alcoholism and to heart failure (Walsh & Levy 2003).

Alcohol is known to have a toxic effect on the heart muscle, changing the subcellular structure and function of the myocytes (Piano & Schwertz 1994). Indeed, a surgical technique to reduce left ventricular muscle bulk in hypertrophy involves alcohol ablation – destroying cells with alcohol. It is not known how much or what types of alcohol are likely to have this effect but it is estimated to be at least ten years of excessive drinking (Fabrizio & Regan 1994). Dose of alcohol and exposure over time, influenced perhaps by genetics, are probably the most significant variables. There are also thought to be metabolic and haemodynamic consequences for the heart with chronic excess alcohol consumption. If a patient with alcoholic cardiomyopathy drinks large volumes of alcohol then they are putting haemodynamic stress on their heart, and as the heart is already weakened this may be enough to trigger acute cardiac decompensation.

Patients with alcoholic cardiomyopathy have dilated hearts. Cardiac enlargement puts the patient at risk of arrhythmias and a sudden onset atrial fibrillation is often the point of referral into cardiology services. In patients with alcoholism there is often associated hypertension and diastolic dysfunction (Fabrizio & Regan 1994). Elevated laboratory liver function tests can help to differentiate a patient with alcoholic dilated cardiomyopathy from a patient with non-alcoholic dilated cardiomyopathy (Wang et al. 1990).

A complicating factor for alcoholics and heart failure is that they often have a very poor lifestyle with regard to diet, sanitation and housing, are likely to smoke and pay little attention to control of risk factors such as high blood pressure, diabetes or cholesterol levels. Alcoholics are highly unlikely to be fully concordant with their treatment. All of these factors contribute to their heart failure prognosis if they continue to drink. Alcoholics who continue to drink have a poor prognosis, whereas alcoholics who abstain can make significant improvements in their functional class and other outcomes (Mølgaard et al. 1990; Teragaki et al. 1993; Spies et al. 2001).

DIABETES

There is a clear link between diabetes and many heart conditions, including heart failure. Until recently there was some controversy over whether a separate pattern of diabetic dilated cardiomyopathy, without other causes of heart failure, existed in some diabetic patients. It is now agreed that diabetics can experience distinct changes in the structure and function of the myocardium by early remodelling and metabolic effects of glycaemia control (Bell 2002; Bertoni et al. 2006). High risk diabetics should have early screening for heart failure and intervention with beta-blockers and ACE-inhibitors even if asymptomatic (Bell 2003).

GENETIC HEART FAILURE

Genetic mutations, either spontaneous or more usually hereditary, are responsible for several disorders of the heart muscle that can lead to heart failure. A lot of research is going into genetics and knowledge is rapidly expanding. It is likely that the prevalence of genetic cardiomyopathies has been underestimated in the past. It is thought that 90 % of hypertrophic cardiomyopathies are familial and 30–50 % of dilated cardiomyopathies have a genetic component (Murphy & Starling 2005). Patients with genetic cardiomyopathies often present at a younger age than other patients with heart failure as a result of either complications or after having been identified through family screening processes after another family member has been diagnosed. These differences mean that their treatment needs may not be the same as for older patients – for example, family planning concerns about genetic inheritance. Genetic Services within the United Kingdom are currently organised on a regional basis.

IDIOPATHIC DILATED CARDIOMYOPATHY

Idiopathic dilated cardiomyopathy is diagnosed when the left ventricle is enlarged and poorly functioning in the absence of ischaemic disease, hypertension or valve disorders.

Gene mutations are recognised as responsible for much of the idiopathic dilated cardiomyopathy. It is probable that some families have specific patterns of cardiomyopathy and some families have a stronger cardiac involvement than others. Is it believed that genetic dilated cardiomyopathy is more widespread than initially thought but current research in this area is not as extensive as for hypertrophic obstructive cardiomyopathy.

HYPERTROPHIC OBSTRUCTIVE CARDIOMYOPATHY

Hypertrophic obstructive cardiomyopathy was first described in 1958 by Teare. Other pseudonyms for the condition include Idiopathetic Hypertrophic Subaortic Stenosis (IHSS), Familial Hypertrophic Subaortic Stenosis, Asymmetric Septal Hypertrophy (ASH) and Disproportionate Upper Septal thickening (DUCT).

It is characterised by an increase in left ventricular wall thickness and a reduction in the left ventricular cavity size; the left ventricle is not necessarily dilated; the septum thickens compared with the left ventricular free wall; abnormal cardiac muscles fibres are short, thick, fragmented and fibrotic. These changes are usually first observed in adolescence.

Clinical presentation is similar to aortic stenosis. Possible symptoms include angina, dyspnoea and syncope; signs may include a jerky, collapsing pulse, prominent apical thrust with a double beat, harsh ejection systolic murmur and a prominent wave in the JVP. Sadly, sudden death can be the presentation.

It is an autosomal dominant inherited condition with specific mutations in affected families, high penetrance and even sex distribution. It is caused by mutation to the genes that code for myrofibrillary proteins. So far at least nine such individual genes with this function have been identified.

The natural history is difficult to predict and although a long life is possible there is a constant risk of sudden death at any age, even in asymptomatic patients. These patients also have a higher risk of bacterial endocarditis. There are no definite helpful prognostic markers although presentation in childhood, syncope and strong family history of sudden death are all worth noting. Non-sustained ventricular tachycardia on monitors is a useful prognostic indicator as in other conditions, as is a failure to have a normal blood pressure response to exercise. Severity of the left ventricular gradient and left ventricular hypertrophy are not significant.

Hypertrophic obstructive cardiomyopathy can be mimicked by other conditions where it is also possible to get a thick walled ventricle without mutation in the myofibril protein genes or disarray of the myofibrils. Other causes include mitochrondrial gene disorders, glycogen storage disease and Fabry's disease.

RESTRICTIVE CARDIOMYOPATHY

Restrictive cardiomyopathy can be either familial or acquired. The genes for the familial pattern have not yet been identified. Acquired restrictive cardiomyopathy in the temperate zones is usually from amyloidosis. In the tropics diffuse perimyocyte fibrosis is a much more common form of restrictive cardiomyopathy (Spyrou & Foale 1994).

Restrictive cardiomyopathy is difficult to diagnose because the left ventricle is almost normal in shape. It does not relax properly in diastole and there can be changes to the echocardiograph reflection. A tissue biopsy is not necessarily helpful because the abnormal tissue is not evenly distributed so there may be false negatives from the biopsy.

ARYTHMOGENIC RIGHT VENTRICULAR DYSPLASIA (ARVD)

Arythmogenic Right Ventricular Dysplasia was first described in 1982 and was thought at the time to be very rare. Since then further studies have suggested it may be responsible for as many as 3–5 % of unexplained sudden cardiac deaths in the under 65s (Marcus et al. 2003).

It is characterised by an area of the right ventricular myocardium being replaced by adipose tissue, with some fibrosis and aneurysmal dilation. It tends to be a small, diffuse or spotty deposition which makes biopsy vulnerable to missing the area and reporting a false negative. Another complication is that a small amount of adipose infiltration into the myocardium is fairly normal, especially in women.

The problem with this small patch of abnormal tissue is that it acts as a substrate for arrhythmias. Arythmogenic Right Ventricular Dysplasia does not usually cause much change in ventricular function. The left ventricle can also be affected in about a third of patients and where this happens the prognosis is poorer (Lemola et al. 2005).

OTHER RARE RAUSES OF HEART FAILURE

As we saw in Chapter 1, there are dozens of possible causes of heart failure and it is beyond the scope of this book to provide details on all of the causes. A few of the rarer causes of heart failure are briefly noted below.

CONGENITAL HEART DISEASE

Congenital heart disease is a complex subject. It is important to note that the end outcome in many forms of congenital heart disease is heart failure. As surgical options have increased and improved outcomes for these patients, more of them are living longer, making heart failure more of an issue for these patients.

PERIPARTUM CARDIOMYOPATHY (PPCM)

Heart failure in pregnancy is rare but potentially very serious and there are occasional maternal deaths as a result of peripartum cardiomyopathy. It can occur before, during and up to a few months after delivery. The most serious is when it occurs during delivery. In the West it occurs in between one in 2400 to one in 15 000 births (Leslie et al. 2004). Maternal mortality can be as high as 50 % (Lampert & Lang 1995).

The mechanisms behind this form of heart failure are not well understood. The left ventricle becomes dilated and hypokinetic. Patients often suffer from acute biventricular heart failure with fluid retention. A postulated mechanism is that it is a form of myocarditis occurring due to the breakdown of the immunological barrier between the mother and the foetus. Another hypothesis is that it is a manifestation of familial dilated cardiomyopathy that becomes apparent with the haemodynamic stresses of pregnancy and birth.

Breathlessness and peripheral oedema are common in normal pregnancy so the diagnosis of peripartum cardiomyopathy can be missed in its early stages.

After recovery it is advised that the mother should avoid further pregnancies in the near future and have close supervision in future pregnancies. Relapse in subsequent pregnancies is not always present. Over half the mothers will not have myocardial damage or long-term chronic heart failure after recovery from the acute phase.

AMYLOIDOSIS

Amyloidosis is a disorder of protein metabolism. It is a systemic disease but can cause heart failure if amyloid infiltrates the heart. This causes a change in the tissues as the amyloid deposits are like fibrotic tissue, which affects the contractility of the myocardium. More particularly, it affects the ability of the heart to relax, with gradual wall thickening and a pattern-like restrictive cardiomyopathy (Parikh & de Lemos 2005).

There are two types of amyloid disease – primary and secondary. The primary sort tends to be more common in younger patients and has a very poor prognosis of less than one year. Occasionally there may be a familial pattern for primary amyloid disease. The secondary type is more common in the elderly and is associated with chronic inflammation. Both types are progressive but primary amyloid disease is the more aggressive condition (Dubrey et al. 1997).

Cases of amyloid heart disease are perhaps underdiagnosed. Signs to look out for are a raised JVP, quiet heart sounds and a low voltage ECG. The echocardiogram may show some areas of brightness. Blood and urine tests are helpful but cardiac biopsy is needed to confirm the diagnosis of amyloid heart failure and this is rarely done in clinical practice. There are no specific medical treatments for the amyloid deposition although chemotherapy and stem cell transplant can be used in primary amyloidosis (Gertz et al. 2005).

SARCOIDOSIS

Sarcoidosis is a systemic condition of unknown cause that can involve the heart in around 20–50 % of cases (Veinot & Johnston 1998). Myocardium is replaced by sarcoid tissue over time. This leads to abnormalities of wall motion and predisposes towards arrhythmias. Treatment is difficult: steroids can induce regression but their use is higher risk in patients with developed heart failure and long term steroid use has been identified as a cause of heart failure in itself (Sekiguchi et al. 1996).

OBLITERATIVE CARDIOMYOPATHY

In obliterative cardiomyopathy a thrombus forms in the apex or inflow segments of either, or both, ventricles. Over time the thrombus converts to fibrotic tissue and a smaller ventricular cavity results.

This form of cardiomyopathy is rare in the United Kingdom but is seen more in tropical countries where nutritional deficiency and ingestion of unknown toxins may be causative factors. This means in the United Kingdom it is more likely to be seen in immigrants from tropical countries than in the native population. It is also sometimes caused by any systemic hypereosinophila such as eosinophilic leukaemia, Churg-Strauss syndrome, Behcet syndrome and idiopathic eosinophilia.

IATROGENIC HEART FAILURE

It is unfortunately possible for heart failure to be induced by medical treatment. Sometimes this is functional, such as too-rapid infusion of a large volume of intravenous fluid causing volume overload and right-sided heart failure. Alternatively, it may be the result of a complication, such as post-surgical bleeding causing acute anaemia and volume deficiency and the heart decompensating with left ventricular failure.

There is also the effect of medications on the heart. Certain drugs are cardiotoxic, such as some chemotherapy agents. Other drugs, such as steroids, NSAIDs and calcium channel blockers, can lead to fluid retention. Drugs will be discussed in more detail in Chapter 10.

CHEMOTHERAPY

Cancer patients who are treated with certain cytotoxic drugs, especially anthracyclines, have an increased future risk of cardiomyopathy (Doyle et al. 2005). This cardiotoxic effect was first described in 1973 but it remains fair to say it is not well known outside of the cancer and cardiac specialisms. The mechanisms are complex but revolve around cellular disruption. Acute cardiotoxicity in the first year after treatment has been suggested to be present in between 5% and 50% of patients depending on cumulative doses of the cytotoxic drug. Chronic effects on the myocardium can be seen years or even decades after the treatment. As cancer treatments are becoming more successful with better outcomes for patients it is likely that greater survival will result in more cases of chemotherapy-induced cardiomyopathy being seen.

4 Outcomes

In this chapter heart failure prognosis, mortality, morbidity and effect on quality of life are discussed. The impact of heart failure is illustrated from different perspectives: that of the patient, their carers, professionals and the health service. The health economic outcomes of heart failure are outlined.

PROGNOSIS

A common question patients ask when told they have heart failure is *'How long have I got?'* Even if patients do not actually express this thought it would be reasonable to expect they would be thinking about it. Even though prognosis is a difficult subject to discuss we have a duty to patients to address it with them. Unfortunately, due to the clinical range of the syndrome, prognosis is a very difficult question to answer honestly and concisely in patients with heart failure.

Giving patients a precise prognosis is impossible because it is affected by many factors, the effects of which are not always fully understood. There are complexities of what type of heart impairment the patient has, the other co-morbidities they may have, their response to treatment and concordance with treatment. For example, we might assume that patients with good systolic function have a good prognosis, but in the CHARMES study moderate or severe diastolic dysfunction was found to be a poor prognostic indicator in hospitalised patients with preserved systolic function (Persson et al. 2007). The single biggest complicating factor is the increased risk of sudden arrhythmic death in heart failure. As more is understood about which patients are at risk of sudden death and more internal defibrillators are implanted, prognosis is likely to change. There are data available on prognosis in different heart failure populations but careful interpretation is needed for the individual patient.

EVIDENCE BASE

Data on prognosis in heart failure comes from surveys, longitudinal studies and clinical trial registries. There are data from the United States and other countries in the developed world but very little from elsewhere in the world.

Box 4.1 Studies of Heart Failure Prognosis

Study	Key mortality results
Hillingdon	• 1 month mortality 19 % • 6 month mortality 30 % • 1 year mortality 38 % • 18 month mortality 43 %
Framingham	• 1 year mortality 43 % men • 1 year mortality 36 % women • 5 year mortality 75 % men • 5 year mortality 42 % women
NHANES-I	• 10 year mortality 50 % men • 10 year mortality 72 % men over 65 • 10 year mortality 36 % women • 10 year mortality 59 % women over 65
Rochester	• Survival similar in 1981 and 1991
Groningen	• 1 year mortality 26 % • 2 year mortality 35 % • 5 year mortality 55 % • 7 year mortality 68 % In a matched control group without heart failure the mortality rates were: • 1 year mortality 3 % • 2 year mortality 6 % • 5 year mortality 20 % • 7 year mortality 30 %
EPICAL	• 1 year mortality 35 %
CONSENSUS	• 10 year mortality 98 %
SOLVD	• 3.5 year mortality 40 % in placebo group • 3.5 year mortality 35 % in enalapril group

From the United States, the Framingham study and NHANES survey give broadly similar results with high mortality and the majority of patients having a prognosis of less than 10 years (Kannel 2000). The NHANES survey noted that mortality was significantly higher in both men and women who were over 65 and had heart failure (Schocken et al. 1992). Both studies also showed that mortality is worse for men, at any age, than for women with heart failure. The gender gap was however not as important as the age gap. The differences in the results between the two studies may be due to the NHANES survey using a wider sample than the Framingham study. A third study from the United States, the Rochester Epidemiological Project, did not find any differences in survival in two cohorts with heart failure taken in 1981 and 1991. The authors suggest that perhaps this reflected that treatments that showed a prognostic benefit in clinical trials were not yet widely used in their samples (Senni et al. 1999).

In the United Kingdom, the Hillingdon Heart Failure study also reported a poor prognosis similar to the results from the United States (Cowie et al. 2000). It showed that a lot of patients died soon after diagnosis – a fifth by one month – illustrating the importance of early diagnosis and initiation of treatments. Other studies from Europe, the Groningen and EPICAL studies, also show a broadly similar pattern for prognosis with around a third of patients with heart failure dying within one year (Van Jaarsveld et al. 2006; Zannad et al. 1999). In the Groningen study older age and male gender were risks factor for worse prognosis, as in the Framingham study results.

Mortality data from the clinical trials are also high. This might be considered surprising as clinical trials usually recruit patients who are younger and have fewer co-morbidities than those in surveys and longitudinal studies; however, clinical trials tend to include a more restrictive definition of heart failure. In the SOLVD clinical trial the mean 42-month follow-up found that 39.7 % of the placebo group and 35.2 % of the enalapril group had died (The SOLVD Investigators 1991). The SOLVD results illustrate clearly that although medications improve prognosis they will not prevent death. In another heart failure clinical trial, CONSENSUS-1, in the 10 year follow-up, of the original 253 patients only five were still alive (Swedberg et al. 1999).

In the studies discussed it is important to note that because of their longitudinal nature, most of the patients were recruited some time ago. They will not, therefore, necessarily have been exposed to the beneficial effects of modern treatments on mortality. If the prognostic benefits shown in the clinical trials of drugs and devices for heart failure are carried through into clinical practise, then future heart failure population studies should show significantly improved prognoses.

PROGNOSTIC COMPARISONS

How does a diagnosis of heart failure compare with the prognosis for other conditions? A study of admissions to Scottish hospitals in 1991 looked at almost 7000 heart failure patients and compared them with 12 000 patients admitted for cancer during the same period. It found that, except for lung cancer, heart failure had a worse prognosis than all types of cancer (Stewart et al. 2001). These comparisons illustrate the seriousness of a diagnosis of heart failure.

The comparison with prognosis in cancer is not straightforward, however. The cancer patient will generally feel reasonably well, with a good level of functioning, until the point of sudden deterioration is reached, usually preceding the terminal stage of the condition. In heart failure, by contrast, the patient often feels unwell from the beginning and their initial level of functioning is often poor. This is followed by periods of rapid deterioration during cardiac decompensation, interspersed with improvements as the decompensation stabilises. This pattern may go on for some time or may be broken by sudden death. Acute heart failure, not surprisingly, has a far worse prognosis than chronic heart failure (Mehta & Feldman 2005). Recognising the terminal stage in heart failure is often difficult for the professionals and the patient – as discussed further in Chapter 12.

When considering prognosis there are various markers that can be used in patients with cancer, including staging and metastases. In patients with heart failure, prognostic markers are less clear. Functional class may seem a good guide – on the principle that the worse the class the more serious or progressive the disease – and there is some trial evidence to support this (Ahmed 2007). However, functional class is a broad guide and can be subjective when dealing with individual patients. Patients' perception of their condition severity is only poorly correlated with clinicians' assessment of NYHA class (Subramanian et al. 2005). Patients with class IV may generally die sooner than those in class II or III but some class IV patients survive many years if they are stable. Biochemical prognostic markers have been studied widely. None is a gold standard but brain natriuretic peptide (BNP) is useful, as it is released in greater amounts the more stress the heart is under. The best marker that is available widely is measures of renal dysfunction such as urea, creatinine and estimated glomerular filtration rate (eGFR). This makes sense, in that if the renal dysfunction is due to poor perfusion then the heart failure is advanced and the treatment is not effective. Having said that, if the renal function is due to primary renal disease it may not be as useful in the consideration of heart failure prognosis.

EXPLAINING PROGNOSIS

When patients ask what their prognosis is it is not very helpful to start listing research studies. Another way has to be found to make the statistics more meaningful. One graphic way to express prognosis is through Kaplan-Meier survival curves – see Box 4.2. When calculated for heart failure they clearly show the serious nature of a diagnosis of heart failure. They can be used with patients as the starting point for a discussion of prognosis. After explaining that the curves are for the heart failure population as a whole there are a couple of positive elements to explain about these graphs: that the curves are improving over time, and that once free of the initial sharp downturn the tail flattens out, meaning that the initial attrition is a lot higher than later on. So if the patient has had the diagnosis for a while then their personal risk is lower. It is also important that these generalised statistics are not applied without contextualising the individual patient. It must be remembered that the average age of patients with heart failure is 76. People who are 76 have a generally shorter life expectancy than younger people and are more likely to have co-morbidities that may reduce their prognosis. In contrast, a younger person, or a patient with no co-morbidity, should generally have a better prognosis than the Kaplan-Meier curve suggests.

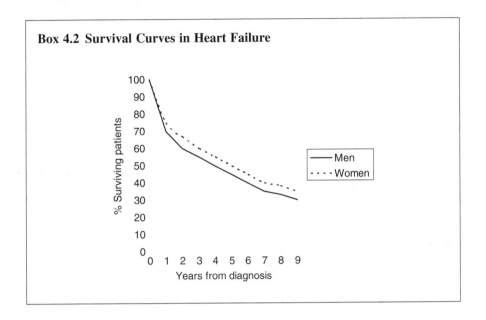

Box 4.2 Survival Curves in Heart Failure

Clinicians are often reluctant to discuss heart failure prognosis for fear of upsetting the patient or their family (Barnes et al. 2006). This reflects that such conversations are difficult and involve advanced communications skills. Explaining a heart failure diagnosis can be seen as an exercise in breaking bad news and the forethought that goes into that process should equally be applied to this situation.

Discussing prognosis will never be comfortable for clinicians, the patient or their family. Ideally, the clinician will have begun to know the patient and their personality as an awareness of what coping strategies the patient may be employing is helpful (Buetow et al. 2001). Open communication is best, avoiding jargon, technical details and clichés, and not making assumptions about either the patient's wishes or about their coping techniques. Sometimes a staged approach can be taken where the topic is introduced early on in the relationship with the patient, ideally soon after diagnosis, and gradually revisited if prognostic markers worsen or the patient shows other signs of deterioration.

The aim is to communicate as simply, explicitly and empathetically as possible. In reality this is difficult, as the answers to questions are often complex, subtle and difficult to convey to a non-specialist. It is the clinician's professional responsibility to reflect on their communication and find ways to explain the situation successfully to all patients and their families. Patients and their families may misinterpret what is said and may choose to focus on certain parts to extract their own meaning.

A good technique is to get people to reflect back what they think has been said, to confirm understanding. Patient and family understanding may also be determined by their personal experiences and previous interpretation of events.

Whilst there is a professional duty to be honest and straightforward with the patient there is also a moral duty to be hopeful. This does not mean saying the patient will get better and be cured – that is not realistic – but it may be possible to reduce symptoms and improve prognosis. Then again, things may deteriorate, either in the short, medium or long term. None the less, even if this happens, the patient can be helped to cope with their condition right up to the end of their life.

Box 4.3 Key Message

Heart failure has a worse prognosis than almost all other medical conditions, but the prognosis is highly variable among individuals and is difficult to predict for individual patients.

MORTALITY

The recording of heart failure as a cause of death varies depending on the registration and coding systems in place. In the United Kingdom heart failure cannot be recorded on death certificates as a primary cause of death, so data from this source is of limited use (Sharpe & Doughty 1998).

MORBIDITY

The interaction between heart failure and other conditions is complex and it is difficult to disentangle causes and effects. What is clear is that patients who have heart failure are also highly likely to have other conditions – for example, they are three times as likely to have ischaemic heart disease and twice as likely to have diabetes mellitus. It is also the case that patients with heart failure who have other conditions are more likely to have a poorer outcome than patients who do not (Thomas & Velazquez 2005).

We will see in Chapter 5 how heart failure with a poor cardiac output puts other organs under ischaemic strain. Multi-organ failure with deterioration of the kidneys and liver is a feature of advanced heart failure and is a poor prognostic indicator.

QUALITY OF LIFE

Quality of life is a conceptual construct that seeks to assess how diseases affect patients. It is influenced by the individual's disease presentation but also by their personality, adaptation skills and health beliefs. Some patients find certain symptoms intolerable while others find the same symptoms bearable; for some patients it is the degree of the symptoms that matters while for others it is feeling a loss of control, fear for the future and lack of cure that are important. When considering quality of life, the effects on social and work relationships are important. Patients adapt to their condition in different ways. Coping is complex and individual. Some coping techniques seem maladaptive to an outsider but it is difficult to criticise or change without a full understanding – for example, some patients might play down the seriousness of their condition as a way of coping in their relations with others (Buetow & Coster 2001).

Quality of life generally deteriorates as heart failure symptoms worsen (Rector et al. 2006). Heart failure is thought to have a greater impact on quality of life than angina, chronic obstructive airways disease or arthritis (Juenger et al. 2002). As an illustration of the complex interplay between cause and effect on quality of life, depression is thought to be present in as many as a third of patients with chronic heart failure and worsens prognosis in all severities of heart failure (Friedmann et al. 2006; Sherwood et al. 2007).

Assessing quality of life is important for a number of reasons. It is known that patients with a poor quality of life are more likely to go to hospital, attend their GP and use other healthcare resources. Quality of life is probably as important a concept as survival for most patients with heart failure. Who wants to live another five years if you can't breathe? Survival is simpler to measure and thus has been looked at as an outcome in more trials than quality of life. Increasing quality of life should probably be seen as the primary goal of treatment in progressive chronic conditions such as heart failure, rather than just increasing survival. Indeed, increasing survival may actually worsen quality of life in some cases.

HEALTH ECONOMICS

Caring for patients with heart failure is expensive. It may inhibit the patient's (or their carers') ability to work. For society there are significant health and social care costs. We will see how patients with heart failure have frequent acute hospital admissions and each of these episodes costs several thousand pounds. The investigations and treatments for heart failure all have a financial cost to the health service. Some costs, such as medicines, are significant and recurrent. Patients with heart failure have frequent contact with community healthcare and often also require social care services, or need to adapt the house in certain ways. The overall cost for patients with heart failure has been estimated at £716 m per annum in the United Kingdom – of which around two thirds are represented by hospital costs (NICE 2003). This percentage is similar in all developed countries.

Hospitalisation rates for heart failure are large and rising. Heart failure was the cause of around 5 % of medical hospital admissions per year in the United Kingdom in the 1990s – greater than the percentage of admissions for myocardial infarctions

(NICE 2003). In the United States, heart failure is the most common admission diagnosis in those older than 65 years (Malki et al. 2002).

Once in hospital the duration of stay is often long. Indeed, the only medical condition with a longer average inpatient stay is stroke. The reason for this lengthy inpatient stay is a complex mixture of clinical factors, co-morbidities and discharge planning delays. Sometimes the lengthy stay is reasonable on clinical grounds: if the patient has had extensive fluid retention then this must be removed gradually. In the United Kingdom the average inpatient stay for heart failure is 11.4 days on a medical ward and 28.5 days on a geriatric ward (NICE 2003). If we think of a typical United Kingdom general hospital having around 250 such admissions per year, then the number of bed days is around 3000. If we then consider each bed day as having a nominal cost of £300, we can estimate that heart failure uses around £1 m of resources per year in that hospital. This relates only to inpatient admissions and does not include any additional investigations, procedures, surgery or outpatient follow-up.

On top of the high cost of initial hospital admission, heart failure patients also have a high re-admission rate. In the United States it is reported that around 40 % of patients admitted with heart failure are re-admitted within six to twelve months (Hamner & Ellison 2005). In the French EPICAL study, 81 % of patients either died or were re-admitted within one year, with the average being two re-admissions in the first year and an average of 27.6 days in hospital (Zannad et al. 1999).

Hospitalisation is the biggest proportion of heart failure costs at present and the most likely to be reducible by service redesign. There are three elements to this: reducing admission, shortening stays and reducing re-admissions. Reducing first admissions is difficult as often this is the first presentation of the condition. None the less, with more community screening and diagnosis it should be possible to recognise people with heart failure earlier and begin treatment in the community. Shortening stays should be achievable where delays to discharge are social rather than clinical, as is often the case. Reducing re-admissions is achieved by better patient education before discharge, appropriate community follow-up and treatment (Moser et al. 2005). If it were possible to reduce heart failure admissions by a quarter, then in a typical hospital the number of bed days would fall from 3000 to 2250. Alternatively, if the length of stay was reduced to 10 days, then the number of bed days would fall to 2500. If both were achieved, then the number of bed days would be halved to 1500. The cost savings for a typical district hospital would be substantial – in the region of £500 000 – and would be enormous if replicated across the country.

Not surprisingly, this is why the Department of Health has a policy focus on cutting admission rates for heart failure. Admission rates are easy to monitor and target. Of course, new presentations cannot be stopped completely so the admission rate will never drop to nothing. If there were savings in the hospital sector it is important to note that some resources would need to be re-allocated to the community to provide support services. The question is, therefore, whether community services are more cost effective than (as well as at being at least clinically equivalent to) those of the hospital.

Box 4.4 Key Message

Heart failure is an expensive condition for the health service but costs can be reduced substantially if patients are managed actively in the community to avoid unnecessary hospitalisation.

---

5 Physiology

In this chapter the physiology of heart failure is outlined with explanations of the structural changes that occur and the functional responses to those changes. The differences between chronic and acute heart failure are presented. This chapter is designed to provide information essential to understanding how heart failure develops and causes symptoms.

THE NORMAL HEART

FUNCTION

The main function of the heart is as a circulatory pump. The right side of the heart receives blood from the venous circulation and pumps that blood to the lungs while, at the same time, the left side of the heart receives blood from the lungs and pumps it around the body.

ANATOMY

Before considering how the heart fails we should familiarise ourselves with the normal structure and function of the heart. The heart has three tissue layers. The inner, endocardial, layer lines the inside of the chambers. The middle layer contains smooth cardiac muscle, known as myocardium, and is the most extensive layer. The fibrous outer layer, the pericardium, covers and secures the heart.

The heart is divided into four chambers to facilitate movement of the blood during the cardiac cycle. On the right side of the heart, deoxygenated blood from venous circulation returns through the inferior and superior vena cava directly into the right atrium. From there it flows through the tricuspid valve into the right ventricle. Then the blood is pumped from the right ventricle through the pulmonary valve into the pulmonary trunk and pulmonary arteries to the lung capillaries, where carbon dioxide and oxygen are exchanged. At the same time, on the left side of the heart, oxygenated blood returns from the lungs through the pulmonary veins into the left atrium. It then flows into the left ventricle through the mitral valve and is pumped from the left ventricle through the aortic valve into the ascending aorta and systemic circulation.

Box 5.1 Diagram of Cardiac Circulation

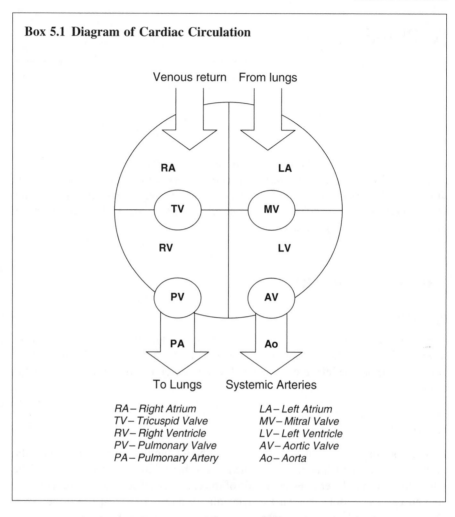

RA – Right Atrium
TV – Tricuspid Valve
RV – Right Ventricle
PV – Pulmonary Valve
PA – Pulmonary Artery

LA – Left Atrium
MV – Mitral Valve
LV – Left Ventricle
AV – Aortic Valve
Ao – Aorta

PHYSIOLOGY

When the heart contracts (systole) and relaxes (diastole), the two sides of the heart are normally co-ordinated to contract simultaneously. The two upper chambers (atria) contract slightly before the two lower chambers (ventricles) in order to facilitate filling the ventricles with blood before their contraction. The process of the movement of blood through the heart is known as the cardiac cycle and each cycle usually takes less than a second to complete.

Box 5.2 Cardiac Cycle

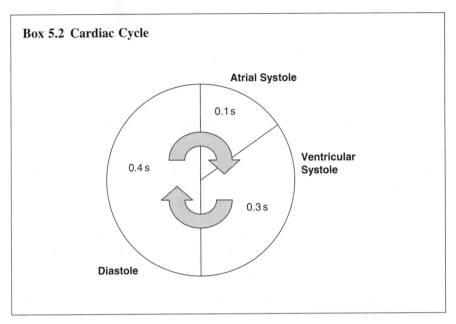

The heart has to supply enough blood to meet the metabolic demands of the body's tissues. The amount of blood it needs to supply will vary – for example, on exercise the demand for blood will be much higher as more toxins need to be removed and more oxygen and nutrients supplied. The heart adjusts to different demands by adjusting its supply through changes to the blood flow (haemodynamics), which are controlled by neurohormonal factors.

HAEMODYNAMIC REGULATION

The body can adjust the flow of blood supply in three ways: firstly, by making changes to the performance of the heart (heart rate, contractility); secondly, by making changes to the *afterload*, the resistance to pumping (blood pressure, systemic vascular resistance); and thirdly, by changes to the *preload*, the pressure within the heart before it pumps – the amount of end diastolic fibre stretch – which is a result of the end diastolic volume (the amount of venous blood return, or plasma volume).

Cardiac output is the amount of blood pumped by the heart in one minute. It is a direct function of heart rate multiplied by stroke volume – see Box 5.3. Heart rate is affected by the autonomic nervous system (sympathetic to speed it up and parasympathetic to slow it down). Stroke volume is the amount of blood in each heartbeat – the pulse volume.

Box 5.3 Cardiac Output

Stroke Volume *multiplied by* Heart Rate *equals* Cardiac Output

$$SV(ml) \times HR(bpm) = CO(l/min)$$

Cardiac Index (CI, $l/min/m^2$) is cardiac output adjusted for body mass

---

Normally, increasing the preload will increase stroke volume and cardiac output. This is because increased preload increases contractility as outlined in the Frank-Starling Law – see Box 5.4. This is a little like the effect of stretching an elastic band – the harder it is pulled the further it will rebound. However, when the muscle fibres are damaged and preload rises then cardiac output can actually be decreased, as if the elastic band has become over-stretched and lost its elasticity – as described by Laplace's Law. It is possible to estimate preload by measuring the pulmonary artery capillary wedge pressure (PCWP) and pulmonary vascular resistance (PVR) using a pulmonary artery catheter but this is rarely done outside of critical care areas.

Afterload is the pressure the heart works against when contracting. It is a resistant force made up of blood pressure, blood volume and blood vessel wall thickness. Normally the left ventricular systolic pressure can overcome afterload without problems but in heart failure this is impaired and a high afterload will reduce cardiac output. It is possible to estimate afterload by blood pressure or systemic vascular resistance (SVR).

Box 5.4 Frank-Starling Law

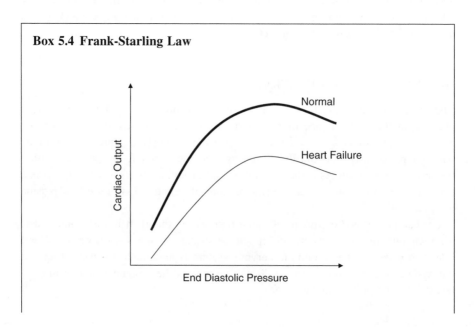

Box 5.4 (Continued)

The Frank-Starling Law describes how, as end diastolic pressure rises, so stroke volume rises on a curve. By raising filling pressures the ventricle is distended and as it is stretched, so contraction is improved. Filling pressure is increased by peripheral vasoconstriction and by increasing the plasma volume. However, increasing filling pressure reaches a plateau on the function curve whereby any further rise in pressure does not increase stroke volume. In the failing heart this curve is flatter – with less stroke volume being achieved for higher end diastolic pressures.

When the heart is distended repeatedly it will dilate and is no longer as mechanically efficient. This over-stretch means the tension required to achieve systolic pressure increases – the Laplace effect – so more energy is expended for each systole.

A dilating heart also changes the shape of the atrioventricular valves leading to regurgitation, atrial dilation and an even poorer function. So high filling pressures in heart failure are a compensatory effect but beyond a certain point they are counterproductive and treatment should be targeted to reduce filling pressures.

NEUROHORMONAL REGULATION

The haemodynamics are influenced by two neurohormonal systems: adrenaline and renin-angiotensin-aldosterone. Activation of these systems is a compensatory mechanism in an attempt to maintain equilibrium and sufficient cardiac output for the needs of the body.

The autonomic nervous system is divided into two parts: the sympathetic and parasympathetic. The sympathetic nervous system, mediated by adrenaline, acts like an accelerator on the heart, and the parasympathetic, through the vagus nerve, acts like a brake. Adrenaline speeds up the heart (positive chronotrophy) and increases the force of contractions (positive inotrophy). This is achieved mainly through stimulation of the beta-adrenaline receptors – beta-1 receptors in the heart. Conversely, within the parasympathetic nervous system stimulation of the vagal nerve will slow down the heart rate and contractility. When the body is under physical (or emotional) stress we need a larger cardiac output – to send more blood to the muscles, heart and brain – so the sympathetic nervous system is activated, adrenaline released and the heart beats faster and harder. This is the primeval 'fight or flight' response.

The second important set of hormones that regulates the heart is that of the renin-angiotensin-aldosterone system. These hormones are concerned with maintaining blood pressure and do so by both direct vasoconstriction and by water and salt retention. When blood pressure falls this is detected in the kidneys and renin is released. Renin activates angiotensinogen, a hormone constantly secreted by the liver, and a cascade follows of conversion to active compounds – see Box 5.5.

Box 5.5 Renin-Angiotensin-Aldosterone Cascade

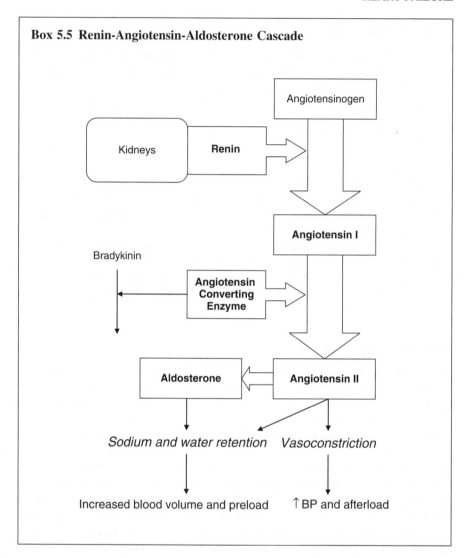

NORMAL EXERCISE RESPONSE

The heart is designed to pump a variable amount of blood to meet metabolic demands. At rest, we might only require three or four litres of blood a minute. On exercise this rises sharply – in athletes cardiac output can increase by a factor of six. The responsiveness of the heart depends on its efficiency. As heart failure means the heart is inefficient it is not surprising that most people with heart failure have no symptoms at rest but only on exertion. This is the rationale behind the NYHA heart failure classification. A patient who is symptomatic at rest is likely to have a cardiac output so poor it is struggling to meet their basic metabolic needs. Conversely, a patient who is only symptomatic at the end of vigorous exercise is able to increase their cardiac output substantially, suggesting the heart failure is well controlled.

In patients with heart failure there are several mechanisms affecting the exercise response. Some are directly attributable to muscle damage – for example, contractility or dyssynchronicity – while others are responses to it, such as heart rate activation and response. Further chronic adverse effects are due to endothelial dysfunction and skeletal muscle changes, as we will see in Chapter 9.

THE FAILING HEART

As we noted in Chapter 1, the heart can fail in a number of ways – on the left side, the right side or both; acutely or chronically; during contraction, relaxation or both; or for structural or functional reasons.

STRUCTURAL ABNORMALITIES

If the structure of the heart is abnormal then the function of the heart may also be abnormal and heart failure may result. Structural abnormalities may either be something the patient was born with (congenital) or something they have acquired. Congenital causes of heart failure include problems with the cardiac valves, abnormal connections or abnormal blood flow between the chambers. Acquired structural abnormalities include some valve diseases, myocardial infarctions, heart muscle fibre abnormalities, hypertension and problems with the blood vessels.

Myocardial infarction is the most common cause of structural abnormality. After a myocardial infarction an area of heart tissue is dead and will not contract – it is *akinetic*. The area around this zone may be ischaemic and not contract well – or *dyskinetic*. This may affect overall contractility of the ventricle and cardiac output. Over time the heart will compensate by enlarging to try to increase stroke volume by the processes noted earlier. This change in shape is known as *remodelling* and unfortunately has a negative effect because of muscle fibre over-stretch. Other problems after myocardial infarction also lead to heart failure, including tears of the chordae tendrae and papillary muscles leading to valve incompetence; ventricular septal defects; and cardiac tamponade – where a rupture occurs from the chamber through to the pericardial sac, leading to a potentially life threatening leakage of blood due to a rise in pressure constricting the heart without any means of dispersal unless there is intervention.

ACUTE HAEMODYNAMIC ABNORMALITIES

Acute heart failure can be brought on by sudden changes in haemodynamics. These are usually caused by major changes in the tissue blood supply or demand – for example, during haemorrhagic or septic shock. Different types of shock may produce different types of acute heart failure. In haemorrhagic shock the cardiac output will fall as the blood volume falls and the heart failure is low-output. However, in septic shock the blood volume will be the same but the demand for blood (to meet the huge metabolic demand of clearing the toxins) will rise and the heart failure will be high-output.

Heart failure may also be precipitated acutely by conditions that lead to excessive preload. Examples of this would be over-administration of intravenous fluids, as this would increase venous return volume, or increased right-sided pressure that may result from reduced contractility as a complication of a right ventricular myocardial infarction. As we have seen, if preload is too high for too long then the muscle fibres will stretch and stroke volume will fall, followed by cardiac output.

Sudden or precipitous hypertension may also trigger heart failure. We have seen how chronic hypertension leads to chronic heart failure. In the case of acute extreme hypertension, high blood pressure means a high afterload and the heart attempts to eject against this, increasing metabolic myocardial oxygen demands and leading to a further reduction in function.

NEUROHORMONAL ABNORMALITIES

As we have seen, activation of the neurohormonal systems is the response of the heart to low cardiac output. Cardiac output is monitored by stretch receptors in the aortic arch and carotid arteries and these trigger activation of the sympathetic nervous system and renin-angiotensin-aldosterone systems. Although this is a normal stress response it is possible for inappropriate or chronic activation of the systems to cause heart failure.

The sympathetic nervous system may be over-stimulated in various ways. It could be caused by severe anxiety, hyperthyroidism or drugs that increase sympathetic activation, such as salbutamol. Conversely, over-blocking of sympathetic action, perhaps by too high a dose of beta-blockers, can cause heart failure. This is the reason why beta-blockers were initially seen as contra-indicated in heart failure, why they should still be introduced cautiously, and may need to be reduced or suspended during periods of acute decompensation.

In severe heart failure there is a chronic depletion of adrenaline hormones in the cardiac nerves. To compensate there is a rise in the amount of adrenaline and noradrenaline in circulation. However, this effect is offset by a gradual reduction in effectiveness and responsiveness of the cardiac beta-1 receptors.

Heart failure is also induced by over-activation of the renin-angiotensin-aldosterone system. Where cardiac output is poor the renal tissues are not perfused and the response is to try and raise blood pressure and retain salt and water to increase renal perfusion. In this case the increased preload leads to dilation of the heart chambers and eventually LaPlace's Law means that contractility and cardiac output is adversely affected.

ACUTE HEART FAILURE

Acute heart failure can occur either as an isolated response to a particular set of circumstances that increases the workload of the heart, such as a severe haemorrhage, or as a consequence of cardiac decompensation resulting from chronic heart failure. Often episodes of decompensation in chronic heart failure can also have a precipitating cause, such as infection or anaemia, but this may not always be apparent. Moreover, what causes decompensation in a failing heart would not necessarily do so in a healthy heart. Indeed, acute episodes are often when the diagnosis of chronic heart failure is unmasked.

Any sudden and significant change in the heart rate or rhythm may lead to acute heart failure, either because the heart cannot adjust or as a consequence of the neurohormonal efforts to compensate. The situation can be complex because chronic heart failure is a cause of increased arrhythmias – through scarring to electrical pathways, ischaemia, a high sympathetic tone, high filling pressures, the effects of muscle stretch and electrolyte imbalances (Baig et al. 1999).

If the heart rate suddenly increases then cardiac output will be too high and high-output cardiac heart failure may occur. To prevent this, stroke volume will have to decrease (in order to maintain the same cardiac output) but reducing stroke volume means a decrease in the fibre stretch. The Frank-Starling mechanism shows that fibres that are under-stretched lose their elasticity. So a tachycardia generally means less contractility. A higher heart rate also means a smaller diastolic filling time, reducing stroke volume, which further exacerbates the situation and leads to the possibility of myocardial ischaemia and angina, as the coronary arteries fill during diastole.

These effects are seen with any tachycardia but where the rhythm is also abnormal the effects are more complex. A chronic arrhythmia such as atrial fibrillation will have negative effects due to unco-ordinated action between the atria and ventricles. This will lead to decreased and turbulent forward blood motion and that will be compensated for by higher atrial pressures. So patients with atrial fibrillation may go on to develop left atrial enlargement and over time this dilation will result in increased atrial pressures being needed to maintain contractility, with a consequence that pulmonary vein pressures may also rise and be transferred back to the lungs, resulting in breathlessness. Any changes in the shape of the left atria and ventricles can also lead to the mitral valve being pulled out of shape and becoming regurgitant, leading to further changes in blood flow and chamber pressures. Another complication is that the turbulent blood flows in atrial fibrillation increase the risk of intracardiac clot formation, which could float off into the blood and become a myocardial infarction, stroke, pulmonary embolism or deep vein thrombosis.

Bradyarrhythmias, such as complete heart block, may also induce heart failure. In these circumstances, as the heart rate drops, in order to maintain cardiac output the stroke volume has to rise considerably, but this may not be possible in an already impaired heart and cardiac output may drop.

Acute heart failure can also be caused by medication. This may either be non-concordance – the patient taking none, too little or too much of their medication – or it may be as a result of inappropriate prescriptions or sudden removal of prescription medication by clinicians. Sometimes this is inadvertent and at other times it is deliberate, where the risks have been considered – reducing medicines to protect renal function, for example.

LEFT VENTRICULAR FAILURE

The left ventricle is the chamber that pumps blood from the heart into systemic circulation. In order to pump the blood it has to operate at high pressures and so it has the largest section of heart muscle, requiring the largest coronary blood supply. This means the left ventricle is the usual site for damage following myocardial infarction.

We have noted earlier how myocardial infarction causes the contractile movement of an area of the heart to be either absent (akinetic) or abnormal (dyskinetic or hypokinetic) and the contraction of the ventricle is impaired. This change in shape may therefore reduce stroke volume. The heart tries to compensate by altering its shape – a process known as remodelling – enlarging (dilation) or building up thicker muscle (hypertrophy). Ventricular remodelling begins at the cellular level with various effects, such as myocyte growth, myocyte function changes, myocyte loss and proliferation and degradation of the extracellular matrix proteins (Baig et al. 1999). The remodelling that occurs after a myocardial infarction is both an early effect of inflammation and a longer process that can go on for months or years. Progression of heart failure is connected to this remodelling and is particularly affected by angiotensin II and noradrenaline.

Remodelling also occurs as a result of long-standing hypertension, even in the absence of myocardial infarction. In this case the pattern is one of concentric left ventricular hypertrophy with increased myocardial mass and probably also diastolic dysfunction. It is also associated with interstitial fibrosis (Baig et al. 1999). Early on patients are asymptomatic although there may be changes on echocardiogram, suggestive of diastolic dysfunction.

Left ventricular function can be judged by the ejection fraction. This is the amount of blood that leaves the left ventricle on systole, as a percentage of the total amount of blood in the ventricle before systole. There is always a residual amount of blood in the ventricle after systole so a normal ejection fraction is around 60 %, as we saw in Chapter 1. In heart failure the ejection fraction can fall as low as 10–20 %. In mild failure the stroke volume is maintained by a compensatory rise in end diastolic pressure. In more severe failure the stroke volume is decreased and the ejection fraction falls.

Box 5.6 Left Ventricular Ejection Fraction

$$\frac{\text{Stroke Volume (SV)}}{\text{Left Ventricular End Diastolic Volume (LVEDV)}} = \frac{\text{Left Ventricular}}{\text{Ejection Fraction (LVEF)}}$$

$$\text{e.g.} \frac{70 \text{ ml}}{120 \text{ ml}} = 0.6 (\text{or } 60\%)$$

In severe left ventricular failure, cardiac output is lowered as the compensatory mechanisms cannot cope. If cardiac output is low the body sends blood differentially to vital organs – such as the heart, brain and muscles – at the expense of the renal, splanchnic and cutaneous vascular systems. This is achieved by sympathetic peripheral vasoconstriction, which maintains arterial pressure. This mechanism is compensatory in heart failure but is clearly bad for the underperfused tissue. It is also maladaptive overall because if arterial pressure is maintained then the failing ventricle has a higher afterload to work against and so is likely to distend more. Incidentally, the differential distribution of blood is worth remembering because it explains why cardiac cachexia (loss of muscle bulk) and symptoms such as confusion are late and worrying signs in heart failure because they are two of the last few areas to lose perfusion, so the rest of the organs are likely to be underperfused too.

If the kidneys are underperfused then the body seeks to expand plasma volume and we have seen how the renin-angiotensin-aldosterone system may also be stimulated by the failing heart. This mechanism can increase plasma volume by up to 30 %. Doing so may be compensatory but if activated chronically this leads to cardiac dilation and the risk of oedema formation as the right side of the heart struggles to cope.

As well as the effect of low cardiac output on circulation, left ventricular failure has an effect on the lungs. Pressure in the pulmonary veins is raised as more blood is pumped to the left to compensate for reduced efficiency, as the right and left heart must pump the same volume of blood. As cardiac output continues to drop the left ventricular end diastolic pressure and pulmonary capillary wedge pressure rise and as pulmonary hydrostatic pressure increases it can overcome the osmotic pressure of the plasma proteins within the blood vessels in the lung. This causes a reversal whereby fluid is forced out of the blood vessels into the lung tissue – known as interstitial or pulmonary oedema. This, along with increased pulmonary hypertension, can cause the sensation of breathlessness in acute left ventricular failure.

RIGHT VENTRICULAR FAILURE

Usually, the right ventricle fails after left ventricular failure – when both fail together it is known as biventricular (or congestive) cardiac failure. This is because as left ventricular failure develops the pulmonary capillary wedge pressure increases, increasing right ventricular workload and oxygen demand.

It is possible to have isolated right ventricular failure. Sometimes myocardial infarctions can affect the right ventricle. The process is the same as for the left ventricle – a localised reduction in muscle contractility and therefore a reduction in the function of the ventricle, with consequent attempts to remodel the ventricle. Other causes of right ventricular failure include primary pulmonary hypertension and valve disease. The most common cause of isolated right ventricular failure is as a consequence of problems with the lungs, such as pulmonary emboli and lung diseases. Where right ventricular failure is as a result of lung disease it is known as *cor pulmonale*.

Right ventricular failure has different symptoms to left ventricular failure. Problems are related to systemic venous congestion. This will be seen as peripheral oedema and congestion of the splanchnic and hepatic systems. Raised pressure within the superior vena cava raises the jugular venous pressure. Raised pressure within the hepatic vein may cause liver congestion, enlargement, nausea and abdominal pain. Raised pressure within the portal vein may cause fluid retention in the abdomen. If there is more volume and pressure within the veins then there will also be a transfer of that pressure to the capillaries. This can be a rise of up to 20–40 mmHg in hydrostatic pressure (the force the fluid exerts against the walls of the blood vessel) when the patient has right heart failure, at the same time that colloid pressure (the osmotic force of plasma proteins holding fluid within the blood vessel) is dropping as low as 7 mmHg due to volume expansion with water diluting the plasma within the capillaries. The net effect is that in right-sided heart failure fluid is forced out of the capillaries and into the tissues, in the characteristic pattern of peripheral oedema.

SYSTOLIC AND DIASTOLIC DYSFUNCTION

The function of the heart can be impaired in terms of either its systolic or diastolic function or a combination of both. Systolic dysfunction is a problem with contraction whereas diastolic dysfunction is a problem of relaxation. This distinction is sometimes not well understood and can lead to misunderstanding. Systolic dysfunction has been regarded as almost synonymous with heart failure and it is perhaps significant that in the GMS contract GPs get points for registering all patients with left ventricular systolic dysfunction (LVSD), yet there is no mention of diastolic failure. This is partly a practical issue – it is much easier to diagnose systolic dysfunction than diastolic dysfunction on an echocardiogram – and partly a result of the fact that diastolic dysfunction is a newer and more controversial diagnosis.

Systolic dysfunction is linked to myocardial contractility and has a direct link to stroke volume and the left ventricular ejection fraction. Contractility is affected by myocardial infarction and hypertension, as we have seen, and systolic dysfunction can either be left ventricular or right ventricular or both.

It has been noted for some time that patients can have a clear clinical presentation of heart failure although their echocardiogram shows preserved systolic function and normal left ventricular ejection fraction. It is now widely agreed that diastolic dysfunction can occur as an isolated phenomenon in around 20–40 % of heart failure patients and is probably more common in the elderly, in patients with renal disease or hypertension, and in women.

The mechanism of diastolic dysfunction is that of a problem with receiving the blood into the heart at rest as the heart does not relax normally. Stiffness is linked to decreased end diastolic volume, shorter muscle fibre length and much higher ventricular diastolic pressure. The result is less ventricular filling and, therefore, stroke volume. Difficulty in relaxing muscles is a result of the take up of calcium and the action of the actin-myosin systems, all of which control contractility. Diastolic dysfunction can be caused by the replacement of normal tissue with scar tissue, such as in myocardial infarction, amyloidosis or hypertrophy.

DILATED CARDIOMYOPATHY

As heart failure progresses the shape of the heart can change as a response – the remodelling process (Baig et al. 1999). The muscle can increase in bulk (hypertrophy) and the chamber might enlarge (dilation).

Hypertrophy can occur either as a primary condition or as a response to hypertension. Left ventricular hypertrophy was present in 44 % of patients in the Hillingdon study and may also be particularly important in people of Afro-Caribbean descent.

Dilated cardiomyopathy is a commonly-seen pattern. The left ventricle is dilated, contracting poorly and the wall thickness is either normal or reduced. The net effect is increased left ventricular mass and chamber size. This increases the risk of apical thrombi and a patient with severe dilated cardiomyopathy is often prescribed Warfarin as a result of this risk. Histologically the myocytes are stretched, lose contractility and become fibrosed or necrotic.

CARDIOGENIC SHOCK

In patients with acute heart failure or severe end-stage chronic heart failure, cardiac output may drop so far that the patient goes into cardiogenic shock. The clinical features are low blood pressure, possible reflex tachycardia, cyanosis, tachypnoea, oliguria or anuria, and possible confusion. Patients in cardiogenic shock have a mortality of over 50 % even with supportive measures to bridge recovery, while without supportive measures cardiogenic shock is fatal.

Box 5.7 Cardiogenic Shock

- systolic blood pressure $< 90\,\text{mmHg}$
- cardiac index $< 2.2\,\text{l/min/m}^2$
- pulmonary capillary wedge pressure $> 15\,\text{mmHg}$
- oliguria then anuria
- cyanosis
- cool extremities
- altered mental state

Part II   Diagnosis and Assessment

6 Clinical Assessment

In this chapter the signs and symptoms of heart failure are presented and their causes explained. The frequency of occurrence of the various signs and symptoms and their diagnostic accuracy is commented on. This is to give the practitioner an appreciation of the clinical usefulness of different symptoms. Variability of presentation is noted as are the differences between acute and chronic symptoms. Particular attention is given to the symptoms suggestive of fluid retention.

ROLE OF CLINICAL ASSESSMENT

Carrying out clinical assessments is a fundamental part of nursing practice. In order to help a patient you must first work out what their health problems and needs are. Clinical assessment can be considered to take place for two purposes in heart failure: firstly, in order to help diagnose patients who are suspected to have heart failure; and, secondly, to monitor progress or assess changes in patients who are known to have heart failure.

Before the widespread use of investigations, clinical assessment was usually enough to diagnose a patient as having heart failure. Unfortunately, as we shall see, the signs and symptoms of heart failure are imperfect as diagnostic tools and no doubt many patients were either labelled as having heart failure when they did not, or not diagnosed as having heart failure when they did. A clinical assessment suggesting heart failure does not mean the patient will have heart failure, as there are many differential diagnoses with similar presentation; conversely, a clinical assessment without any indication of heart failure does not rule out heart failure. Now that investigations can in most cases prove the diagnosis, clinical assessment is used more as part of the screening process – raising enough suspicion that the patient may have heart failure to warrant further investigation.

The second important role of clinical assessment is as a useful tool to monitor a patient's progress and act as an early warning mechanism to detect changes in the patient's condition. It is in this context that most nurses will be using clinical assessment skills – for example, in heart failure clinics or in primary care cardiovascular review clinics. Recognising as early as possible patients who are deteriorating allows for more opportunity to treat that patient.

Box 6.1 Role of Clinical Assessment

Diagnosis
To raise suspicion of heart failure and trigger request for diagnostic investigations.

Review
To assess if the patient is deteriorating

Worsening cardiac output
Fluid retention

To assess if further complications or treatment side effects.

ASSESSMENT SKILLS

Assessing patients with heart failure is sometimes difficult and at other times easier – depending on factors such as how the condition is affecting the patient, how acutely unwell they are, whether they can articulate their condition and whether the patient is already known to the clinician and they therefore have a baseline assessment of that patient to compare against. Influencing all of these is the skill and experience of the clinician making the assessment.

A patient with acute decompensated congestive heart failure and who attends the Accident and Emergency department with severe dyspnoea, orthopnoea and anxiety, with tachycardia, badly swollen legs and lung crepitations will immediately have heart failure recognised as the most probable diagnosis. An overweight patient at home with exertional breathlessness and lethargy, cool limbs and a weak pulse may not as readily raise concern about heart failure.

At its most basic level clinical assessment is an appreciation of when a patient is ill. For patients in the community, educating them and their relatives to recognise the early signs and symptoms of cardiac decompensation and fluid retention, so that they can ring for help and have treatment adjusted, is vital for keeping them out of hospital. A nurse who sees the patient regularly will also have good insight into whether their condition is different to normal.

Patients can be instructed to weigh themselves regularly. Sudden weight increases are characteristic of fluid retention and are usually the first sign of this – before ankle swelling or increased breathlessness. As a rough guide, 2 kg of weight gain within a week for an average sized woman and 3 kg for an average sized man is a rapid enough weight gain to be of concern. Weighing is easily done in the home and has the additional benefit of involving the patient in their own monitoring, giving them a degree of control over their condition, which can be psychologically helpful. For patients who struggle to interpret or act on weight gain an option may be to use a telemedicine weighing system, which involves an interactive set of scales that transmits the patient's weight through the telephone system back to a designated clinician.

When assessing patients' symptoms it is easy enough to learn the checklist of heart failure symptoms. More skill – in both communication and consultation – is needed to draw those symptoms out and to place them in a coherent context. For example, a patient who is labelled as having paroxysmal nocturnal dyspnoea but who does not have orthopnoea, may not actually have paroxysmal nocturnal dyspnoea but may in fact be having panic attacks.

Examining patients rarely provides information not already suspected from their history but it is useful as part of completing the picture. For example, a history of increased breathlessness, recent ankle swelling and orthopnea may make the clinician suspect fluid retention; examining for signs of peripheral fluid retention can help to confirm this. The training, experience and skill of the clinician dictate what information can be gained. The measurement of heart rate and blood pressure is probably the simplest and most valuable information. More advanced examination skills are valuable for nurses when they are working autonomously.

None of the assessment skills are outside of the scope of nursing. To argue so would be to argue nurses cannot operate autonomously or without direct supervision and this is clearly disproved by experience in many areas of practices, including heart failure. That is not to say that in order to carry out a full and competent assessment, additional training is not required. Unfortunately, basic nurse training is not adequate for this purpose. A heart failure nurse should be an advanced practitioner as well as a specialist nurse.

PRESENTING COMPLAINT

It is valuable to find out why the person has sought help at that time. Has a symptom just started? Has an existing symptom become intolerable? Has a partner insisted they get seen? Information on how long a condition has gone on for and what is the nature of the problem is important. Equally important is finding out the patient's perspective. This may differ from the concerns of the clinician. Any mismatch between the two perspectives may be an explanation for issues of treatment concordance.

Box 6.2 Typical Presenting Complaints in Heart Failure

- breathlessness
- fatigue
- difficulty in sleeping
- ankle swelling

PAST MEDICAL HISTORY

We have noted in Chapter 3 that heart failure is not a disease in itself but is a syndrome caused by a variety of underlying conditions. It is important to try and work out any cause in order to treat it, or at least to reduce its effects. The clues to the underlying cause of the heart failure will lie in the patient's medical history.

Heart failure should be suspected in any patient with a history of myocardial infarction. It is not always clear if a patient has had a myocardial infarct and unfortunately the lay term of 'heart attack' is imprecise and open to misunderstanding. Most patients will know if they have had a heart attack but bear in mind that some patients think they have had one when in fact they have had it mentioned – but not necessarily confirmed – as a potential diagnosis when they had chest pain. Indeed, some patients say they have had dozens of heart attacks. Occasionally patients will assume they have had a heart attack because their symptoms were similar to that of a relative or friend who had a heart attack. Also, occasionally a patient will say they have had a heart attack when in fact they had an acute arrhythmia. It is useful to find out if it was a confirmed diagnosis: how and by whom – a hospital specialist diagnosis after investigations is likely to be more accurate than a retrospective GP diagnosis made on history alone. Remember that the patient may not have been aware they have had a myocardial infarct as sometimes these are 'silent' – i.e. without symptoms – especially in diabetics, the elderly and in women.

A history of hypertension is always important to consider in heart failure. Hypertension is almost always silent so it is often only found during screening as part of age-related reviews or another medical examination. A patient who says they do not have high blood pressure should be asked when last they had it checked. If the patient does have hypertension then the length of time they have had it should be determined, if known, as well as whether they have been on treatment and if this has controlled their blood pressure. A long history of hypertension is more closely associated with heart failure than a shorter history (Kannel and Belanger 1991).

While taking their medical history, note other medical conditions that may lead to heart failure, either in themselves or as a result of the treatment. Rheumatic fever leading to cardiac valve disease may lead to heart failure. Patients who are taking long term steroids or other anti-inflammatory agents may develop heart failure. Chemotherapy can lead to heart failure in some cases.

Box 6.3 Important Medical History in Heart Failure

- ischaemic heart disease

    myocardial infarctions
    angina
    revascularisation

- hypertension
- arrhythmias
- valve disease
- rheumatic fever

LIFESTYLE REVIEW (SOCIAL HISTORY)

Checking the cardiovascular risk factors for heart disease – diabetes, hypertension, obesity, smoking, high cholesterol and family history – is important. This is not just because of the close link with ischaemic heart disease but also because these factors often independently predispose towards heart failure. For example, poorly-controlled diabetes leads to a particular form of global cardiomyopathy, as does alcoholism. As some forms of heart failure are due to inherited cardiomyopathies, family history is important to consider, especially in patients presenting at younger ages. A family history with sudden and unexplained deaths should raise suspicion of cardiac involvement.

Finding out about patients' social circumstances is also vital as part of the treatment planning process. For example, if someone's partner is a smoker, then the patient is far less likely to be able to stop smoking than if they are not (Park et al. 2004). If a patient does not cook their own meals then any dietary changes are going to have to be discussed with the person who does. Some lifestyle issues – such as income and housing – might be important for the patient's health but may need the involvement of other agencies to resolve.

Box 6.4 Cardiovascular Risk Factors and Social History

Risk factors

- smoking
- hypertension
- diabetes mellitus
- high cholesterol
- diet
- obesity/inactivity
- family history of premature CVD in first degree relative

Social history

- inactivity
- diet
- salt
- alcohol
- smoking
- housing
- stairs
- mobility
- income/work/benefits
- carers

MEDICATION REVIEW

Looking through the patient's prescription is invaluable. It will help to confirm any medical history the patient has already mentioned and suggest others the patient has not mentioned either through forgetfulness or because they consider them irrelevant to their heart condition. It also may indicate some medicines that may exacerbate heart failure. For example, effervescent painkillers contain a great deal of salt, while NSAIDS and some calcium channel blockers can also lead to fluid retention. The timing of the prescription is also worth noting as sometimes changes to timing can have an effect on symptoms or tolerability. Most important of all, and not to be taken for granted, is concordance – if the patient is not taking their medicine then they definitely will not work.

Medicines are discussed in greater detail in Chapter 10.

SYMPTOMS OF HEART FAILURE

Heart failure is usually suspected due to the presence of certain symptoms. Some symptoms, such as exertional breathlessness, are regarded as classic for heart failure. Other symptoms, such as fatigue, are equally common but perhaps less well recognised as due to heart failure. Unfortunately, many symptoms are difficult to ascribe to exact causes and it is important to remember that symptoms may have multiple causes or causes that are not due to heart failure.

It is also important to remember that not all patients with heart failure have symptoms – either because their heart failure is mild or because it is well controlled. Although the majority of patients with heart failure will have symptoms, the absence of symptoms does not rule out heart failure.

When taking the patient's history it is useful to know which symptoms are the most closely linked to heart failure – or how accurate they are for diagnosis. Various studies have considered the helpfulness of signs and symptoms in heart failure and these are summarised in Box 6.5.

A similar pattern emerges from these studies for all the symptoms: low sensitivity but better specifity. In other words, the symptoms are poor at indicating people who have heart failure but are also unlikely to point to someone as having heart failure when they do not. Subgroup analysis in one study suggested diagnostic accuracy was lower for these symptoms in the elderly and in women (Harlan et al. 1977). None of the studies has a strong positive predictive value so their usefulness in diagnosis must be treated with caution. That does not mean symptoms do not have an important role to play in reviewing patients: someone who is chronically mildly breathless but suddenly becomes acutely breathless has had a significant change.

Box 6.5 Studies of Signs and Symptoms of Heart Failure[*]

Study Author	Size	Methods	Signs/Symptoms
SOLVD (Drazner et al. 2003)	N = 4102	Subgroup analysis of accuracy of signs of heart failure in mild left ventricular systolic dysfunction	JVP; third heart sound
EPICA (Fonseca et al. 2004)	N = 1058	Study of the diagnostic accuracy of signs of heart failure in Primary Care	JVP; ankle oedema; lung crepitations; third heart sound; tachycardia
Ahmed et al. 2004	N > 1000	Retrospective chart review in 11 Alabama hospitals	Rest dyspnoea; exertional dyspnoea; orthopnoea; paroxysmal nocturnal dyspnoea; fatigue; ankle oedema
Badgett et al. 1997	N = 817	Study of signs and symptoms of heart failure in four GP practices in Devon	Exertional dyspnoea; JVP; ankle oedema; lung crepitations
Davie et al. 1996a	N = 259	Study of the diagnostic accuracy of signs and symptoms of patients admitted to hospital with suspected heart failure	Tachycardia; JVP; third heart sound; murmurs; crepitations; wheeze; ankle oedema; displaced apex beat
Harlan 1977	N = 1306	Study comparing signs and symptoms of heart failure with evidence of left ventricular ejection fraction of < 40 % on angiogram	Dyspnoea; orthopnoea; paroxysmal nocturnal dyspnoea; ankle swelling; tachycardia; lung crepitations; third heart sound; JVP

Minimum of 250 patients in studies
JVP = jugular venous pressure

Assessment is the collation and interpretation of data. While individual symptoms may lack accuracy in isolation it is logical this will increase in combination. In other words, if a patient has rest dyspnoea, orthopnoea and paroxysmal
nocturnal dyspnoea, they are much more likely to have heart failure than if they only
have rest dyspnoea. In one study the presence of three or more symptoms – from
exertional dyspnoea, rest dyspnoea, orthopnoea, paroxysmal nocturnal dyspnoea,
increased weight and ankle oedema – raised positive predictive value to above 90 %
(Ahmed et al. 2004).

Box 6.6 Symptoms of Heart Failure

- breathlessness

  at rest
  on exertion
  suddenly from sleep (paroxysmal nocturnal dyspnoea)
  when lying flat (orthopnoea)

- wheeze
- cough
- haemoptysis
- fatigue
- poor exercise tolerance
- ankle swelling

SHORTNESS OF BREATH (SOB)

The sensations of difficulty in breathing (dyspnoea) and shortness of breath (SOB)
are classic symptoms of heart failure. Breathlessness due to heart failure can be
either chronic or acute. Patients with heart failure may be breathless with or without
excess fluid retention.

Not all breathless patients have heart failure. Indeed, a minority of all breathless
patients will have heart failure. Other common causes of breathlessness include
respiratory disease, obesity, anaemia and endocrine diseases (Struthers 2000). It is
also possible to have heart failure but to be breathless from another cause such as
a chest infection. In order to work out whether the cause of the breathlessness is
heart failure the symptom needs to be explored in detail using questions such as
those in Box 6.7.

Box 6.7 Questions about Breathlessness

- For how long have you been breathless?
- When did it start?
- Did it start suddenly or slowly?
- Are you breathless all of the time?
- Are you breathless at rest?
- Do you have to stop while climbing the stairs?
- Does walking uphill make you breathless?
- What activities/exercise make you breathless?
- How far can you walk before becoming breathless?
- Are your exercise levels deteriorating?
- Is your breathlessness getting worse?
- Do you get breathless when upset?
- Are you breathless when lying down?
- How many pillows do you use and why?
- Do you wake up suddenly at night feeling breathless?
- If you are breathless at night, what helps to relieve this?
- Do you have a cough? If so, dry or wet? Colour and volume of sputum?
- Does anything make your breathing worse?
- Does anything make your breathing better?
- Are some days worse than others?
- How does if affect your life?

Breathlessness is a physiologically complex symptom and there are probably several mechanisms causing this in patients with heart failure (Coats 2001). Psychological factors should also not be overlooked as higher levels of depression, fatigue and lower health perception scores have been shown to contribute to dyspnoea (Ramasamy et al. 2006).

Exertional breathlessness is a normal physiological reaction. As we exercise, cardiac output has to rise to meet metabolic demands and lung ventilation has to match the increase in lung perfusion: failure to do so results in breathlessness and a switch to anaerobic metabolism. At the same time, exercise increases venous return, increasing pulmonary congestion and stimulating the fine nerve endings around the terminal alveoli, so causing the sensation of breathlessness. There is a variation in exercise threshold among people, dependent on their gender, body shape, age and fitness level. Once exertion stops, demand drops and is swiftly matched again by supply, hence the breathlessness eases once exercise stops.

In patients with heart failure the ability of the heart to supply the increased demand during exercise is impaired, so the exercise threshold is reached earlier, with increasing breathlessness. Research shows that in patients with chronic heart failure abnormalities in peripheral circulation also contribute to shortness of breath on exertion and fatigue (Coats 2001).

Patients with severe heart failure can be breathless at rest. This may be either because of very poor cardiac output or due to chronic pressure changes stiffening the lungs and bronchial walls, which interferes with airflow. This can cause a wheeze – sometimes rather confusingly known as *cardiac asthma*. There is also the possibility that patients with rest dyspnoea may be breathless due to fluid retention or acute decompensation. In one hospital study rest dyspnoea had a high sensitivity but low sensitivity for diagnosing heart failure – in other words, rest dyspnoea as a symptom was present in most patients with hospitalised heart failure but rest dyspnoea was also present in a lot of patients without heart failure (Ahmed et al. 2004). If the patient does have acute heart failure then other signs and symptoms will be present as well as breathlessness. Often patients will have been told that they have 'fluid on the lungs' if they are seen during acute heart failure. Whilst this may be true at the time, it is often misunderstood by patients to be an explanation as to why they are chronically breathless, which can lead to coping problems later as they assume they must still have fluid on the lungs.

When assessing the patient with heart failure and breathlessness, especially if the pattern or severity of the breathlessness is changing, it is worth looking for factors that may be contributing to the problem. The most likely would be common problems such as chest infections and anaemia. A chest infection can provoke heart failure due to increased haemodynamic demands or by the formation of pleural effusions. Anaemia makes breathlessness worse because there is less haemoglobin for oxygen to bind to and be transported by.

It is worth bearing in mind that breathlessness is more likely to be due to lung problems rather than heart problems. Lung diseases are very common, especially chronic obstructive lung diseases. Complicating matters is the fact that many patients with heart failure may also have lung disease. Spirometry is useful in building up a picture as to whether the breathlessness is predominately cardiac or respiratory. When exertional breathlessness was placed in the context of a carefully taken medical history in a study of 146 patients, the symptom had a diagnostic accuracy of 74 % for heart failure (Schmitt et al. 1986).

Patients who are breathless often assume they are short of oxygen and that if they were given oxygen the breathlessness would improve. In fact most patients with heart failure and breathlessness are not hypoxic. Giving them oxygen therefore will not help – a patient who is fully oxygenated with complete haemoglobin binding cannot increase the amount of oxygen delivered (unless it is by increasing the small amount of oxygen dissolved in plasma, but this requires hyperbaric pressures). It is possible that giving oxygen to these patients may be harmful as oxygen is a vasoconstricting agent. The exceptions, when the patient is hypoxic and oxygen may help, is if the patient has acute heart failure with pulmonary oedema or if they have lung disease. In acute heart failure, if the patient has pulmonary oedema, then they may be hypoxic because of lung congestion. In this case oxygen can help while definitive treatment – morphine, diuretics and nitrates – removes the excess fluid and lowers preload and afterload. Frequently patients will assume it is the oxygen that has helped improve their breathlessness and this can lead to them wanting to continue on oxygen long term. The problem with having oxygen long term is that of psychological dependency and the impact it has on social functioning, as becoming oxygen dependent means the patient becomes virtually housebound.

Another possible mechanism of dyspnoea that is sometimes overlooked, and yet is common in inactive heart failure patients, is obesity. Obesity is associated with breathlessness on the simple level of reducing the capacity of the lungs to expand and increasing the workload of the organs. Specifically, obesity may decondition the heart, result in fatty infiltration of the myocardium and lead to altered filling pressures. In one large study obesity was not associated with left ventricular systolic dysfunction but was associated with ventricular remodelling and increased left ventricular end diastolic pressure, which suggests diastolic dysfunction (Powell et al. 2006).

ORTHOPNOEA

Some patients with heart failure become breathless when they lie flat. This is known as orthopnoea. The question to ask the patient is how many pillows they use under their head at night – they will usually need three or more if they have orthopnoea. Of course, some patients sleep upright for reasons of comfort – for example, those with arthritic problems. To differentiate orthopnoea, a follow-up question to ask is what happens if the patient slips down the bed? If they answer that they suddenly become breathless then it is orthopnoea they are describing.

The physiological mechanism that causes orthopnoea is not completely understood but it is thought to be caused by pressure changes and the effects of increased venous return to the heart when the patient is lying flat. It is a temporary symptom as sitting up eases the effect.

As a symptom orthopnoea is more specific to heart failure than breathlessness, especially when the two are present together. Orthopnoea should not occur in healthy individuals and isn't usually present in patients with respiratory disease.

Generally orthopnoea only occurs in people with severe heart failure and tends to be a fairly late symptom. So the absence of orthopnoea will not rule out milder heart failure. Remember also that the use of medications, especially those such as diuretics and nitrates, which reduce preload and fluid retention, means a patient who might have suffered from orthopnoea may now not be suffering from it. This is a good illustration of how, when taking a history, it is important to ask not just about present symptoms but also about those that the patient may have had prior to treatment.

Orthopnea is likely to be a worrying and troublesome symptom for patients. Symptoms that occur at night tend to be more disturbing and there are also clearly practical difficulties if the patient is sharing their bed with someone. Sometimes patients will prefer to sleep upright in a chair rather than go to bed. Although this may seem sensible most chairs are not designed to sleep in and patients may develop back problems as a result.

There is no simple cure for orthopnoea. If the patient is orthopnoeic as a result of cardiac decompensation then treatment may relieve the problem. If the orthopnoea is chronic then this may not be possible and instead it may be necessary to focus on adaptation, by getting a bed that can be raised at the head.

PAROXYSMAL NOCTURNAL DYSPNOEA (PND)

Paroxysmal nocturnal dyspnoea is the sensation of sudden breathlessness occurring at night. Classically the patient will report waking suddenly and feeling breathless, an hour or two after having gone to bed. This is often accompanied by feelings of anxiety. It is also sometimes associated with clear or whitish sputum – occasionally pinkish or with blood streaks. Copious frothy or blood-speckled sputum is more common in patients with pulmonary hypertension. Paroxysmal nocturnal dyspnoea occurs in severe heart failure and is thought to be due to pressure changes in a failing heart related to position and venous return. Typically the symptom will last for up to twenty or so minutes and is relieved by the patient standing or sitting upright with their feet out of bed. When exploring the symptom sometimes the patient will describe gasping for air at an open window.

Like orthopnoea, paroxysmal nocturnal dyspnoea is a more specific symptom of heart failure than breathlessness alone. Paroxysmal nocturnal dyspnoea tends to be a symptom of severe or acute heart failure and is not likely to be present in well-treated patients or patients with milder forms of heart failure. As diagnostic symptoms, orthopnoea and paroxysmal nocturnal dyspnoea have poor sensitivity but better specificity – they don't occur in many patients with heart failure but when they do occur the patient is likely to have heart failure.

To make clinical assessment more difficult, paroxysmal nocturnal dyspnoea can easily be confused with nocturnal panic attacks. These panic attacks usually also last for 10–20 minutes but are more likely to leave the patient with a feeling of dissociation and unease. Panic attacks will make the patient anxious and breathless, sometimes sweating heavily or feeling nauseous. Panic attacks at night may have links with sleep patterns and they seem more common during periods of REM sleep, especially in the hours before dawn.

Paroxysmal nocturnal dyspnoea is a symptom that often occurs during acute decompensation. In that case the symptom should vanish once the heart is stabilised. If the patient continues to have chronic attacks of paroxysmal nocturnal dyspnoea it can be very distressing for them. Sometimes changes to the timing of medications are helpful – for example, moving a nitrate to night-time. GTN spray can be used during episodes of paroxysmal nocturnal dyspnoea to provide some relief, as it will reduce preload. Being given permission to use GTN also gives a sense of control back to the patient and makes them feel less helpless. Along the same lines, waking at night feeling unwell is distressing and it can help to have a clear plan if this happens: for example, the patient should be advised to swing their legs out of the bed, to breathe more deeply and slowly, and then to use their GTN spray. For chronic or persistent paroxysmal nocturnal dyspnoea attacks, sometimes relief can be gained by raising the head off the bed a few inches. This is postulated to reduce venous return and lower the preload pressure.

PERIPHERAL FLUID RETENTION

Fluid retention is a classic symptom of heart failure. It occurs due to fluid being retained as part of the neurohormonal mechanisms to compensate for poor cardiac output (Jackson et al. 2000). This extra fluid leaks out into the tissue spaces due to hydrostatic pressure and osmotic processes, as we saw in Chapter 5. Fluid ends up in the ankles due to gravity, hence its alternative name of *dependent oedema*. In a bed-bound patient the fluid will build up around the sacrum. If the fluid continues to build up then the level it is observed at will rise and eventually include the genitalia and abdomen.

Detecting fluid retention can be difficult in the early stages but eventually it becomes unmissable. The sooner it is detected the sooner treatment can be initiated, the less unwell the patient will become and the lower the risk for the patient. The first thing that happens when fluid is being retained is that the patient's weight will increase. This is because water is absorbed quicker than food and most of the body is made up of water. It is possible for weight to increase suddenly and dramatically. We will discuss weighing in the next section. Patients who do not weigh themselves may still be aware of their weight increasing. It is advisable to ask them to look out for feeling heavier, bilateral ankle oedema, genital oedema, abdominal swelling and difficulty in zipping trousers up and putting their shoes on.

Ankle swelling is the most common symptom of peripheral fluid retention. Unfortunately, ankle swelling is very common at the end of the day even for people in normal health or if they have been standing for long periods. It also happens more frequently to elderly people and occurs in a range of diseases involving infection and inflammation, such as lymphoedema, cellulitis and liver and endocrine diseases. So further information is needed when considering ankle swelling. If the swelling is a result of heart failure it will be bilateral. Unilateral swelling by definition must be a problem localised to that particular limb and is not indicative of a systemic condition such as heart failure. The swollen ankle will be soft and pitting to pressure – leaving a blanched indentation for several minutes after pressure is removed. In contrast, lymphoedema tends to be hard and non-pitting to pressure. Fluid tends to accumulate around the ankle and top of the foot. To make a distinction, ask the patient if they have trouble getting their shoes on. Looking for marking from socks is not foolproof as the socks will mark the legs if they are too small or the elastic too tight. Ankle oedema from heart failure may eventually seep out through the skin as a fluid leak, but this is unusual. Weeping legs are more common in other chronic swellings such as lymphoedema or cellulitis. Ankle swelling from heart failure generally will not cause discoloration unless there is also poor peripheral perfusion. Of course, it is possible to have heart failure and poor peripheral circulation simultaneously; however, this is an important difference as removing excess fluid will not necessarily improve chronic poor circulation, so the legs may be slim but discoloured.

Swelling higher up in the body is unusual in mobile heart failure patients but it can occur. Genital swelling, particularly scrotal in men, can be severe in acute fluid retention. There are of course many differential diagnoses so the context is important, such as whether or not the genital swelling is accompanied by ankle swelling and increased breathlessness.

Ascites is the collection of free fluid in the abdominal cavity. For the patient, this feels like bloating and there is often visible distension. There are many alternative causes of abdominal distension − often beginning with the letter F: fat, faeces, foetus or flatulence, as well as fluid. There are various ways to differentiate these from fluid and this will be discussed in the section on examination (pages 81–3).

FATIGUE AND LETHARGY

Probably the most widely experienced symptoms of heart failure are exertional fatigue and general lethargy. They are also symptoms that can be very debilitating for patients and make a significant difference to their quality of life.

Fatigue and lethargy are very common findings in a variety of conditions and also as a normal variant within healthy people. This means there are many differential causes and their value as diagnostic symptoms is limited. When they do occur they are also very hard to ascribe with certainty to heart failure. It is important not to assume the symptoms are due to heart failure but to consider other causes − such as anaemia and depression − that may be treatable.

The cause of fatigue in heart failure is probably multifactorial and both physical and psychological causes should be considered. Reduction of the blood supply to skeletal muscles is an important factor (Jackson et al. 2000). This can be addressed through exercise training programmes.

The effects on activities of daily living should be discussed: some people may describe the fatigue as terrible but they may still be managing, while other people may be struggling and need help. Also consider how the patient is coping − some strategies may be maladaptive, such as getting into a cycle of doing less because of fatigue and then being able to do less because of deconditioning. A common presentation with fatigue is for the patient to describe good and bad days. It is useful for patients to know this is common and that a good response is, where possible, to plan activities for certain weeks rather than specific days, thus reducing their frustration. Knowing that it is simply part of the medical condition can also give the patient permission to have a bad day. Knowing the symptom can be managed is often liberating and gives hope.

SLEEP DISTURBANCE

Many patients with heart failure have difficulty sleeping (Wolk et al. 2005). There are of course many reasons why a patient may have difficulty in getting to sleep or staying asleep for a restful amount of time. Insomnia is a common finding in the general population, especially as people age, and also in conditions such as depression, which are more common in heart failure patients. As a symptom of heart failure, sleep disturbance is common but it is far too unspecific to be useful diagnostically.

It is thought that sleep disturbance in heart failure may be due to changes in diurnal rhythms due to abnormal cotisol release (Erickson et al. 2003). At other times it is due to unpleasant nocturnal symptoms, such as paroxysmal nocturnal dyspnoea. Some medications, notably beta-blockers, have been linked to sleep disturbance. Fatigue may cause patients to sleep during the day and feel less sleepy at night.

Sleep apnoea has also been associated with heart failure, in particular with left ventricular systolic dysfunction. The converse is not true; not all patients with sleep apnoea have heart failure. A complicating factor is that sleep apnoea is associated with obesity and obesity is common in heart failure patients. There is some evidence that sleep apnoea is associated with severity of heart failure and is an indicator of poor prognosis (Merritt 2004). This may be due to sleep apnoea in heart failure being responsible for chronic sympathetic nervous system activation, hypertension and arrhythmias (Dincer and O'Neill 2005; Floras 2005).

Patients with heart failure and sleep apnoea can benefit from nocturnal oxygen though either continuous positive airways pressure (CPAP) or non-invasive positive pressure ventilation (NIPPV) devices. Anecdotally, some patients report great benefits from these and they have been used in some small trials with varying effects. The evidence base is however not strong or clear and NICE have made no recommendations as yet beyond that further research is needed (NICE 2003).

SEXUAL DYSFUNCTION

It is common for patients with heart failure to have problems with sexual function. As you might expect, these are difficult topics for patients to discuss and the true level of these problems may well be under-reported. If a patient does mention it they will likely do so at the end of the consultation but that does not mean it is an afterthought for them. More likely they have been building up courage and they know that by mentioning it at the end their embarrassment will be limited by the end of the consultation.

There are several reasons for sexual dysfunction in heart failure patients: the condition itself, the treatments and the psychological consequences of the condition. Heart failure reduces peripheral circulation and this includes the sex organs. We have seen how patients may also be breathless on exertion and may be chronically fatigued. Patients may also be taking many drugs that affect blood pressure, such as ACE-inhibitors, or that seem to reduce libido directly, such as beta-blockers.

It is worth differentiating whether the patient is reporting loss of libido or sexual function, or both, as these may respond better to different treatments. Specialist referrals may be necessary but will be dependent on what is available locally – urologists and counsellors can be helpful. Sexual dysfunction in heart failure is discussed further in Chapter 8.

PALPITATIONS

There is an association between heart failure and arrhythmias, which the patient may report as symptoms of palpitation, dizziness or blackout (syncope). Arrhythmias, especially ventricular arrhythmias or paroxysmal fast atrial arrhythmias, may cause acute heart failure due to haemodynamic stress. Arrhythmias are also a consequence of chronic heart failure if the shape of the heart is stretched, as in mitral regurgitation and left atrial enlargement (Watson et al. 2000).

The symptom of sudden loss of consciousness, syncope, should not be ignored. In heart failure, patients who have syncope are more likely to have sudden death (Middlekauff et al. 1993). Episodes of syncope or near-syncope should be the trigger for further investigations: an ECG and bloods in the first instance, probably an echocardiogram, then perhaps specialist testing such as a tilt table or electro-physiology studies.

OTHER SYMPTOMS

The list of potential symptoms associated with heart failure is large. This is because any organ that is underperfused will lose function and eventually fail. So, a patient with renal failure secondary to heart failure may have a reduction in urinary volume (oliguria) or even absence of urine (anuria). Anaemia is both a symptom and a cause of heart failure. If the gastro-intestinal tract is underperfused the patient will absorb less food and may become cachexic, or nausea may become a prominent symptom.

Depression and anxiety are common symptoms in patients with heart failure. Psychological and behavioural factors have been shown to play a significant role in rehospitalisations (Moser et al. 2005). Some authors have hypothesised that poor perfusion of the brain can lead to cognitive functional impairment (Lackey, 2004). Like fatigue, this is a difficult symptom to definitively ascribe to heart failure, as some cognitive impairment is common anyway as people get older.

SIGNS OF HEART FAILURE

It would be very helpful if there was a clinical sign that told you that patients either had heart failure or they did not, when a patient is examined. Unfortunately, no such sign exists. However, there are a large number of clinical signs associated with heart failure – see Box 6.8.

Clinical signs may seem more objective to assess than symptoms – they are observed directly by the clinician rather than told to the clinician by the patient, but there are several issues that make signs less reliable. Accuracy and consistency can vary among clinicians (*inter-observer variability*) who are looking for signs (Ismail et al. 1987). A sign may be judged to be present when it is not, or vice versa. Naturally, these issues are more important if the sign is an unusual or subtly presenting sign. A second problem is the reliability of the link between the sign and heart failure. This is the diagnostic accuracy. As with symptoms, when looking for signs of heart failure it is important not just to collate the data but also to interpret it, to ask whether a coherent pattern is emerging and if the signs make sense alongside the symptoms reported.

It would be helpful to know if some signs are more important in heart failure assessment than others. Studies have looked at the diagnostic accuracy of the signs of heart failure and these are summarised in Box 6.5. It is important in this context to note that many of these studies were of hospitalised patients and will be of a more severely affected cohort who are more likely to have signs that are clearer. In a less differentiated cohort, for example in a community diagnostic heart failure clinic, the accuracy of the signs is likely to be lower. This caution is supported by a study that found clinical signs of heart failure in primary care had a high false positive rate (Remes et al. 1991).

It has been questioned whether the presence of signs of heart failure may be useful in detecting asymptomatic patients with heart failure. An analysis of the SOLVD study looked at this question in a cohort of 4102 patients with asymptomatic or mildly symptomatic heart failure (Drazner et al. 2003). This found that the relative risk of heart failure was 1.38 (95 % confidence interval 1.09 to 1.73, $P = 0.007$) if a third heart sound or raised JVP was present. Finding these signs in an undiagnosed asymptomatic patient should therefore lead to investigations for heart failure.

Box 6.8 Signs of Heart Failure

- changes in pulse (rate, regularity, character and volume)
- changes in blood pressure
- raised JVP
- displaced apex beat
- third heart sound
- gallop rhythm
- bilateral pitting ankle oedema
- ascites
- scrotal oedema
- sacral oedema
- wheeze
- lung crepitations

PULSE

In Chapter 4 we saw that the purpose of the heart is to pump sufficient blood to match the changing demands of the tissues. Cardiac output has to vary and to achieve this either the heart rate must change or the amount of blood in each heart beat – the stroke volume – must change. The heart rate will increase or decrease and it is usual in healthy individuals for the heart rate to vary from around 40 beats per minute (usually seen at rest or sleep) to over 100 beats per minute (usually during exercise, although also possible if emotionally stressed).

We noted how, in heart failure, cardiac output drops and compensatory mechanisms are activated. On the one hand, the body tries to increase stroke volume by increasing intravascular volume and myocardial contractility. On the other hand, the heart increases its rate. Tachycardia is therefore a sign seen in cardiac decompensation. As a response mechanism tachycardia is maladaptive in patients over time as the faster the heart beats the less diastolic filling time there is, as well as less volume and filling pressure in the ventricles, less myocardial fibre stretch and reduced contractility. Furthermore, the coronary arteries are filled during diastole, so the higher the heart rate the more chance of coronary ischaemia.

There are many causes of tachycardia and it is always an abnormal finding at rest. Sinus tachycardia is seen as a response to the increased metabolic demands of infection and thyrotoxicosis, both of which may precipitate heart failure. A tachycardia may be indicative of a change in rhythm so the regularity should be checked (using a large artery, such as the carotid) and an ECG requested if any irregularity is detected.

Slower than normal heart rates – bradycardias – are also abnormal and should be followed up. If the heart rate is slow enough then it is possible for patients to be put into heart failure. The usual causes of slow heart rates are heart blocks and these become more prevalent in the elderly. The other important causes of bradycardia are iatrogenic medication effects, particularly with beta-blockers and digoxin (Kernan et al. 1994).

Irregularity in the heart rate may be a normal variant – either through sinus arrhythmia or ectopy – or may indicate an arrhythmia. Atrial fibrillation, as both a cause and consequence of heart failure, is present in about a third of patients with heart failure (Watson et al. 2000).

The nature of the pulse is less easy to assess than its rate and regularity. None the less there are some potential findings. Pulse volume is a crude reflection of left ventricular stroke volume. It is often reduced in heart failure. Detecting this manually is difficult. Pulse alternans, a succession of large then small volume beats, is seen in severe left ventricular dysfunction. It is easily confused for coupled ventricular ectopics. A characteristic jerky pulse is seen in patients with hypertrophic cardiomyopathy with a left ventricle outflow tract obstruction, including aortic stenosis.

BLOOD PRESSURE

The body adjusts blood pressure automatically in order to maintain perfusion to all the organs and the peripheries. In heart failure both high and low blood pressure are seen.

Long-standing high blood pressure, we have noted, is a cause of heart failure. If a person has heart failure it is important that their blood pressure is brought within acceptable levels as soon as possible otherwise the processes causing the damage will continue. The current Joint British Societies' guidelines (JBS2) recommend a blood pressure below 140/90 or 135/85 in diabetics (British Cardiac Society et al. 2005). Achieving this can be a challenge as blood pressure tends to rise with age and high blood pressure can be very resistant to treatment in some individuals.

If a person is in acute heart failure, sometimes high blood pressure is seen. This is part of the neurohormonal compensatory mechanisms the body deploys. This is the body tightening the peripheral arteries to increase peripheral vascular resistance, thereby increasing venous return to try to maintain stroke volume and cardiac output. None the less it is maladaptive and causes acute left ventricular failure and lung pressure to rise, leading to breathlessness and pushing fluid into the interstitial tissues in the lungs and congesting the alveoli. Reducing the high blood pressure with a diuretic, nitrates and morphine is an urgent treatment goal in these cases. Eventually in acute heart failure the blood pressure may drop very low as the compensatory mechanisms fail and the patient goes into cardiogenic shock.

Patients with heart failure may also develop low blood pressure. This can be indicative that the heart is not pumping powerfully. Often, low blood pressure occurs as a consequence of heart failure medications. ACE-inhibitors, angiotensin receptor blockers, nitrates, beta-blockers and diuretics all lower blood pressure.

If the patient has blood pressure that is too low, then organs may be under-perfused and start to lose function. It is difficult to be certain how low is too low for blood pressure and it varies from person to person depending on their body size and blood pressure history. A systolic blood pressure below 80 mmHg is almost certainly too low. A blood pressure reading of between 80 and 90 mmHg systolic may well be acceptable as long as the person has no symptoms, such as dizziness or excessive fatigue, is not dehydrated and shows no signs of organ damage. A systolic blood pressure above 90 mmHg will be adequate for most patients.

Like heart rate, indeed like all the assessments, value often lies in repeat assessments providing a rounded picture of the patient so that any changes from their norms can be detected and investigated.

FLUID RETENTION

The signs of fluid retention come in two patterns: those that indicate peripheral oedema and those that show pulmonary oedema. Peripheral oedema is a result of right-sided or biventricular heart failure whereas pulmonary oedema is due to left ventricular failure. It is possible to have either or both.

Box 6.9 Signs of Fluid Retention

Peripheral

- weight increase (more than 2–3 kg in a week)
- bilateral pitting ankle/leg oedema
- genital oedema
- ascites
- raised JVP

Pulmonary

- lung crepitations
- basal dullness

A sudden weight increase is usually the first sign of fluid retention. This is because water is absorbed quicker than solids. A patient will know their weight has increased if they weigh themselves regularly. They may also feel heavier and sometimes may find trousers or skirts suddenly tight. Our weight does alter during the day and over time so it is difficult to know what weight increase is a sign of fluid retention. A guide increase of around 2 kg (5 lb) for an average-sized woman and 3 kg (7 lb) for an average-sized man within a week is about right.

Pitting ankle oedema can be examined by using firm pressure behind the medial malleolus for ten seconds (it is easy to palpate the posterior tibia artery at the same time to check peripheral circulation). If a blanched indentation is left in place for some time after release then pitting ankle oedema is present and by working up the leg it is possible to determine how high the fluid is.

Ascites can be checked in a number of ways. Firstly, look for the shape and position of the abdominal distension. Fluid should produce a uniform shape dependent on gravity. The technique of shifting dullness is relatively straightforward. This involves percussing the distended abdomen until the tone changes. This indicates where fluid changes to gas (gas is lighter than fluid and will rise). Mark the point and move the patient onto their side and repeat. If fluid is present then the point at which the percussion tone changed will have moved position. Another technique to hear free fluid is the succussion splash whereby the abdomen is rocked to try to detect free fluid splashing against the abdominal wall or passing as a wave under a hand placed on the patient's side.

In patients who are suffering from fluid (or pressure) overload the pressures within the right side of the heart increase. This is reflected in the right sided central veins and can be visualised in the jugular venous pressure (JVP) because it connects directly to the right atrium without any intervening valves. In health the JVP is barely visible flickering over the clavicle in patients positioned at 30–45 degrees. If the patient has fluid or pressure overload then the JVP will rise and the vein become distended. It may even fill all the way to the earlobe. So measuring the

JVP gives additional information as to whether there is right-sided heart failure and fluid retention. Conversely a low JVP means that there is too little volume or pressure – for example, if the patient was dehydrated. As a sign of heart failure the JVP has low sensitivity and specifity. This is partly because of the effects of lung disease causing pulmonary hypertension. Also there is a high degree of inter-observer variability in measuring this sign (Cook 1990; Seth et al. 2002) and poor accuracy compared with invasive gold standard measurement of right atrial pressures (Davison & Cannon 1974).

The mechanisms for pulmonary oedema are different to peripheral oedema as they involve pressure changes in the lungs as a result of left ventricular failure. Raised left atrial pressure is reflected back to the lungs and capillary hydrostatic pressure increases until it overcomes the osmotic pull and fluid is forced out from the capillaries into the lung tissue spaces. This fluid will tend to collect lower down the lungs and in both lungs. To detect this fluid, auscultation of the lungs may reveal extra noises such as crackles in both bases. These can become coarser and higher in more severe cases.

Unfortunately, testing for lung crepitations is not a very specific test for heart failure. In a study assessing 207 elderly patients with acute dyspnoea, lung crepitations were absent in 35 % of cases where they were expected and present in 29 % of cases where no cause was evident (Connolly et al. 1992). Another study found that lung crepitations had poor predictive accuracy for heart failure if that was the only sign present but if other signs or symptoms were also present then sensitivity rose to 81 % and specifity to 47 % (Gillespie et al. 1997). If present, lung crepitations should be placed in context as they can occur in many other conditions – for example, chest infections. Like heart failure patients, smokers will also be breathless. If pulmonary oedema is suspected it is best confirmed by chest X-ray.

Patients who have both peripheral and pulmonary oedema are showing signs of both right- and left-sided heart failure with decompensation and are therefore in congestive heart failure.

SIGNS OF STRUCTURAL CHANGE

There are various signs that give an indication that the structure of the heart has, or is, changing in response to heart failure. These findings are useful in both diagnosing heart failure and considering prognosis.

Touching the patient's chest may reveal the apex beat, thrills, heaves and thrusts. The apex beat is the point at which the patient's heartbeat is felt most strongly when the chest is palpated. Sometimes a displaced apex beat occurs in heart failure. In this case the apex beat is likely to be displaced down and laterally. This is as a result of the heart increasing in size (Eilen et al. 1983). Normally the cardiac apex beat is felt in the fourth or fifth intercostal space just lateral to the mid-clavicular line on the left side. It may be visible or felt as a pulsation in thinner patients. The apex beat is not, however, palpable in up to half of the patients (O'Neill et al. 1989) so if you cannot find it, don't worry. Thrills are palpable murmurs and are most commonly a result of mitral or aortic stenosis in adults. If a thrill is detected by palpitation, a murmur on auscultation will be present. A heave felt (or even seen) at the lower sternum may indicate right ventricular hypertrophy and a sustained thrust felt at the apex might indicate left ventricular hypertrophy or mitral regurgitation.

Cardiac auscultation might reveal several abnormalities associated with heart failure. In severe left ventricular failure the mitral valve cusps move close together at the start of systole and the first heart sound can be quiet. If the right ventricle is impaired then right ventricular pressure can rise and the closing of the pulmonary valve be delayed – this will lead to increased normal splitting of the second heart sound. A similar splitting of the second heart sound occurs in right bundle branch block. Alternatively, the second heart sound may be reverse split – with the pulmonary sound being heard before the aortic sound – caused by delayed left ventricular systole due to left bundle branch block or severe left ventricular systolic dysfunction. A third heart sound (S3) is abnormal except in young people. If accompanied by a tachycardia this sometimes sounds like a distinctive gallop rhythm. It is thought this occurs as a result of increased left atrial pressure and also occurs with mitral regurgitation. One small study found the third heart sound was highly predictive of an ejection fraction of less than 50 % when present, but that absence of the third heart sound was not uncommon with patients with milder heart failure (Patel et al. 1993). Inter-observer variability is a major problem with detecting the third heart sound (Joshi 1999).

Heart murmurs may indicate a problem with the blood flow through the heart. Usually this would be a problem with a valve. As we have seen, this may either be a cause or a consequence of heart failure. This distinction will influence whether the patient will be helped by surgical intervention on the valve.

Box 6.10 Signs of Chronic Heart Failure

- displaced apex beat
- heaves
- third heart sound

SYSTEMIC SIGNS

There are various changes that occur as a consequence of heart failure and that may produce signs throughout the body. These are rare unless the heart failure is severe.

The hands and face are the sites of a large number of potential signs. Anaemia is common in patients with heart failure. Sometimes it is seen acutely but more commonly as a chronic condition and is associated with renal dysfunction (Anand et al. 2005). It may be seen in the skin colour and pallor of the mucous membranes. Cyanosis may also be seen in the fingers and mucous membranes and can indicate poor gas exchange as a result of heart failure. Generally patients with heart failure will not be hypoxic but they can become hypoxic during acute decompensation or if the chronic heart failure is severe or complicated by lung infarctions or disease. Finger clubbing may be seen in chronic heart failure but as it is also seen in chronic lung, liver and endocrine disease it is not very helpful diagnostically in differentiating heart failure. Cholesterol deposits may be visible as xanthoma, xanthelasma or corneal archus. Although not directly implicated in heart failure there is a clear link with coronary heart disease and therefore with myocardial infarction and heart failure.

An abdominal examination can also reveal signs that are relevant in heart failure. Patients with heart failure in its severe form often lose their appetite and have problems with food absorption as the blood supply to their bowel decreases. This can lead to cardiac cachexia. Look for loss of muscle bulk, particularly in muscles like the thighs and deltoids. Hepatic enlargement may occur due to venous congestion in right-sided and biventricular heart failure. In this case, the JVP should also be elevated. An expansive and pulsating liver occurs in patients with severe tricuspid regurgitation, which can occur with a failing right side of the heart. Patients with heart failure and liver dysfunction also sometimes report abdominal tenderness over the liver.

ASSESSMENT TOOLS AND COMPETENCY

There are different models and tools available to facilitate clinical assessments, some of them specific to heart failure – such as the Framingham Chronic Heart Failure Diagnostic Criteria (Schellenbaum et al. 2004).

Competency in clinical assessment can only be achieved through suitable training, practice and experience. In the United States nurses have achieved advanced practice through accredited clinical masters' programmes for the past 50 years. In the United Kingdom training and education for clinical assessment is unfortunately often more *ad hoc*. In the United Kingdom there has tended to be a greater emphasis given to specialist rather than advanced nursing practice. Whilst heart failure assessment requires an in-depth cardiac knowledge it is important that other systems, such as respiratory, can be assessed as well by the clinician.

It is important to be able to elucidate the symptoms in a meaningful way and integrate them with the examination findings. The examination is less important than the history and should be focused to rule in or rule out hypotheses that have arisen from thinking about the history. If the history and examination do not match up there is something not quite accurate in either the data or its interpretation. One simple way to try and differentiate and collate the assessments of heart failure patients during a review is to consider whether they are 'wet' or 'dry' (are they retaining fluid) and whether they are 'cold' or 'warm' (is the cardiac output very poor) – see Box 6.11. Using this conceptual model has the advantage of allowing you to think more clearly about what treatment is needed and how high-risk the patient is at that time.

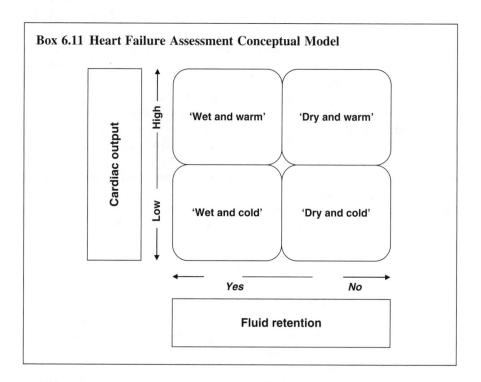

Box 6.11 Heart Failure Assessment Conceptual Model

It is possible to use a tick box protocol for assessment. As we move onto electronic systems this is becoming more prevalent, especially in primary care. The advantage is that consistency and enabling warnings can be built into the pathways and software if electronic. There are also disadvantages, however, especially if poorly designed – for instance, straight jacketing the data and the thinking process, and leading in the wrong direction. Another disadvantage is a false sense of security.

Whatever system is used it is important to have a permanent record and a record that is accessible for comparing with previous ones. An advantage of dedicated heart failure services is that the same practitioners will tend to see the patients repeatedly and are therefore more likely to recognise any changes from the patients' normal condition.

Box 6.12 Assessment Checklist

History

- presenting history
- past medical history
- surgical history
- social history
- cardiac risk factors
- medication history
- symptom review

Examination

- hands
- arms
  radial pulse
  lying and standing blood pressure
- head and neck
  JVP
  carotid pulse
- thorax
  apex beat
  heaves and thrills
  heart sounds
  airways
  lung sounds
- abdomen
  obesity
  ascites
  liver size
- legs
  pedal pulses
  ankle oedema
  peripheral circulation

7 Investigations

This chapter outlines investigations used in the assessment of patients with heart failure. The value of the information potentially gained from different investigations is explained. Normal ranges and how they change in heart failure are noted. The strengths and weaknesses of the various investigations are considered. Some notes are also made on cost effectiveness and service delivery of different investigations.

USE OF INVESTIGATIONS

Investigations are essential to the diagnosis and management of heart failure. A diagnosis of heart failure can be suspected from the clinical assessment but can only be confirmed by investigations (NICE 2003). They can also help to demonstrate the cause of the heart failure and how the heart failure has developed. Finally, they can be useful as a guide to progress or to assess deteriorations.

It is worth remembering that investigations are overused in many medical conditions (Winkens & Dinant 2002). There are obvious cost implications to using many investigations – each echocardiogram, for example, costs between £50 and £100. The more patients are referred for investigations, the more pressure will be placed on the services providing these investigations, which means that either capacity will need to be increased by employing more staff and buying more equipment, or supply should be limited through a waiting list. Lack of capacity and high demand has traditionally been an issue with echocardiogram services. It is also important to remember that sending a patient for an investigation has an effect on the patient and their carers – their expectations and anxiety are raised as they await the results. For all of these reasons investigations should be used in a controlled and thoughtful manner in which the results will help diagnosis or affect treatment.

Box 7.1 Uses of Investigations

- to confirm the diagnosis
- to rule out the diagnosis
- to define the problem
- to detect significant changes

INVESTIGATIONS FOR DIAGNOSIS

A clinical assessment will have raised the suspicion that the patient has heart failure, as we saw in Chapter 6. The patient may be experiencing symptoms such as exertional breathlessness or signs such as ankle oedema. Their history might reveal a previous myocardial infarction or years of high blood pressure. A clinical assessment may show whether left- or right-sided heart failure, biventricular failure and fluid retention are present. We have also noted that if heart failure is acute or

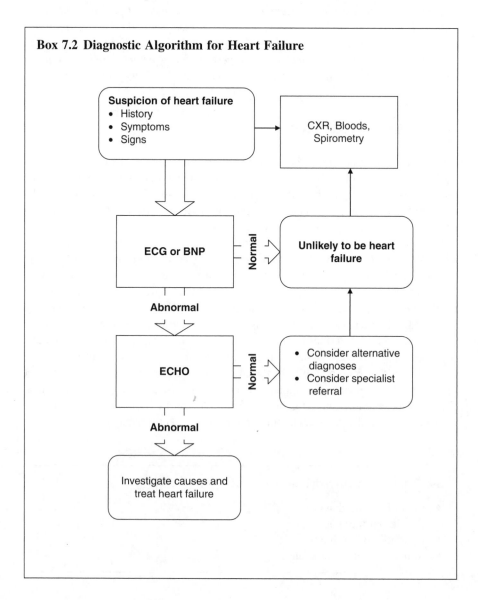

Box 7.2 Diagnostic Algorithm for Heart Failure

Suspicion of heart failure
- History
- Symptoms
- Signs

CXR, Bloods, Spirometry

ECG or BNP

Normal → **Unlikely to be heart failure**

Abnormal

ECHO

Normal →
- Consider alternative diagnoses
- Consider specialist referral

Abnormal

Investigate causes and treat heart failure

severe the signs and symptoms will be easier to see but when the heart failure is chronic and either moderate or mild then the possibility arises of a misdiagnosis from the clinical assessment. Unfortunately, a clinical assessment is not accurate enough to provide a definite diagnosis of heart failure.

In order to confirm a diagnosis of heart failure, further investigations are needed. The NICE guidelines provide a clear framework for this by recommending that patients have either an electrocardiogram (ECG) or a brain natriuretic peptide (BNP) blood test. These tests have a high negative predictive value for heart failure: if they are normal then it is highly unlikely the patient has heart failure and other causes of their symptoms should be considered. If either of these is abnormal then the patient might have heart failure and should have an echocardiogram done. The echocardiogram represents the diagnostic gold standard for systolic heart failure but it is worth remembering that it is not as powerful a tool to identify diastolic dysfunction.

Other investigations may also be required depending on the individual patient's presentation. Because there are a number of underlying causes and presentations, the scope of the supporting investigations will vary. It is likely that as part of the diagnostic process most patients will require at least a full set of relevant blood tests and a chest X-ray. Patients with a background of possible ischaemic heart disease, suggested by either their history or ECG changes, should go on to stress testing and coronary angiography, if appropriate.

Box 7.3 Examples of the Diagnostic Accuracy of Investigations for Heart Failure

Investigation	Study	Sensitivity	Specificity	PPV	NPV
ECG	Houghton et al. 1997	89%	46%		
	Davie et al. 1996a	94%	61%	35%	98%
	Fonseca et al. 2004	81%			75%
BNP	Januzzi et al. 2005	90%	84%	70%	98%
CXR	Fonseca et al. 2004	57%			83%
Echo	Crawford & Henry 1997	93%	32%	75%	66%

INVESTIGATIONS FOR FOLLOW-UP

Once the patient has a diagnosis of heart failure then the question of how frequently further investigations are needed arises. Clearly, an important consideration is whether the patient is stable or not. An unstable patient is likely to have frequent changes to their treatment and therefore blood tests may be required regularly. A patient who has become unstable may need investigations to look for the causes of their deterioration – such as thyroid function tests, a full blood count, renal or liver function tests or chest X-rays, depending on the clinical assessment. For a stable heart failure patient a minimum of six-monthly blood tests is suggested in most clinical guidelines, in order to detect any chronic deterioration early on.

The question of how often to repeat the echocardiogram, or even if there is any justification to do so, is unclear. If the patient's condition has worsened it may well be warranted, especially if there is concern over possible problems with the cardiac valves. Over-use of echocardiograms can lead to some patients becoming anxious about the results and fixating on measures such as the left ventricular ejection fraction. As a general rule it is best only to request investigations if the results are likely to change the treatment.

HEART FAILURE SCREENING

We have seen in Part I how heart failure is very common and a major public health concern. We also noted that some patients are more at risk than others. In Part III we will discuss how early treatment is more effective clinically and in terms of cost than waiting until the patient is poorly. This combination of factors is also seen in other medical conditions, such as cancers, and has led to interest in screening programmes.

If more screening was carried out on asymptomatic high-risk patients, then undoubtedly more patients with heart failure would be detected. This would have the benefit of allowing earlier intervention. Whether this sort of screening would be economically viable is unclear (McDonagh 2002). Such a screening programme, it could be argued, might also lead to more patient anxiety and labelling with chronic disease.

Even if screening was not considered for a wide population in the future there is still likely to be more screening for heart failure of targeted individuals whose family histories suggest potential genetic cardiomyopathy. There is increasing evidence that genetic cardiomyopathies are under-diagnosed at present.

There is also the question of who would manage any screening programmes. Most of our knowledge relates to a secondary care environment but it is questionable whether existing hospital-based services could cope with the increased workload of a screening programme. By the same token, it is known that primary care has had barriers to diagnosing and managing heart failure in the past in terms of suitable equipment and staff resources (Fuat et al. 2003).

ELECTROCARDIOGRAM (ECG)

The electrocardiogram is an essential investigation tool for patients with heart failure. It is a graphical representation – with time measured along the x axis and energy on the y axis – of the summation of electrical activity emanating from the heart. The ECG provides a good deal of information about the structure and function of the heart: the heart rate is confirmed; the rhythm of the heart can be established and any abnormal rhythms diagnosed; and the shape of the ECG complexes can give indications of structural defects within the heart and previous myocardial infarctions.

RESTING 12-LEAD ECG

A standard 12-lead ECG uses 10 electrodes (four bipolar and six unipolar) to give 12 views of the heart's electrical energy at different positions on the body surface. The advantage of using different views is that any abnormalities located at a particular region of the heart, such as hypertrophies and infarctions, can be seen.

A 12-lead resting ECG is a quick, low-cost investigation that can be carried out in any setting that has a machine and a suitably-trained member of staff. Interpretation takes a little more skill but is not as difficult as it may initially appear: a structured analytical approach helps and there are several excellent courses and books available. Most ECG machines also have diagnostic software built into their systems, which is useful as a check but should not be relied on to provide a definitive diagnosis as they are not necessarily entirely accurate (Davie et al 1996b).

The disadvantages of ECGs are that they provide relatively limited information which is only truly valid for the period of the recording. For example, heart rate varies continuously depending on the condition of the heart and the demands being placed on it, while arrhythmias are sometimes paroxysmal – they come and go. Other information, for example the pathological Q waves seen after some myocardial infarctions, is likely to be permanent. Wherever possible, it is helpful to have previous ECGs from the same patient to compare against.

As an investigation for heart failure, the ECG is very helpful as a normal ECG virtually rules out left ventricular systolic function. A normal ECG makes heart failure unlikely but an abnormal ECG does not confirm heart failure (Davie et al. 1996a). A systematic review of the diagnostic accuracy of the ECG in heart failure found that the majority of studies had similar results, reporting sensitivity of greater than 80 % with lower specificity (Davenport et al. 2006). For this reason ECGs are recommended as the initial investigation in patients who are suspected of having heart failure.

There are a large number of abnormalities that may show up in the ECG of a patient with heart failure. Abnormalities of heart rate may be seen, as both bradycardia and tachycardia can be either a sign or a consequence of heart failure. There may be abnormalities in the heart rhythm, common examples of which would be heart blocks, intraventricular septal conduction delays and atrial arrhythmias. Evidence of previous myocardial infarctions, such as pathological Q waves or poor R wave progression, may be present. There could be indications in the shape of the complexes – such as large voltage QRS complexes, downward-sloping ST segments and T wave inversion – that the chambers of the heart are hypertrophied. It has also been suggested that low voltage complexes in patients with heart failure are a marker for poorer prognosis (Kamath et al. 2006).

Box 7.4 Potential ECG Abnormalities in Heart Failure

Rate

bradycardia (HR < 60)
tachycardia (HR > 90)

Rhythm

sinus tachycardia
atrial fibrillation or flutter
non-sustained ventricular tachycardia

Conduction delays

heart blocks
left axis deviation
left or right bundle branch block

Complex morphology

pathological Q waves
poor R wave progression
large voltage QRS, downward sloping ST segment and T wave inversion
low QRS voltages

As well as being useful in diagnosing heart failure, ECGs may help at various later stages. If there is a concern, perhaps during examination or as a result of new symptoms, that the patient's heart rhythm may have changed – for example, from sinus rhythm to atrial fibrillation – then an ECG is indicated. The new development of classic cardiac symptoms such as palpitations, dizziness or blackouts should always be followed up with an ECG and then a longer period of monitoring, such as a 24-hour ECG, as required.

Abnormalities found on the ECG will influence treatment. A patient with fast atrial fibrillation will need the rate controlled (as the faster the heart beats the less time it has to fill with blood) and anti-coagulation (as an irregular rhythm leads to turbulent blood flow and increased risk of blood stasis and clot formation). Patients with heart blocks may need a pacemaker and patients with heart failure and intraventricular conduction delays may be suitable for cardiac resynchronisation therapy using biventricular pacemakers.

AMBULATORY ECG MONITORING

A small tape cassette-sized monitor, attached to the patient with electrodes, is used to take an ambulatory ECG. It stays on for a set period of time, such as 24, 48 or 72 hours, and makes a continuous recording. The patient is usually also asked to fill in a diary sheet recording any abnormal symptoms or significant events and the time they occurred. The recording is downloaded and analysed along with the diary sheet.

Being able to monitor a patient's heart rate and rhythm over a longer period can be useful in patients with heart failure. This is particularly the case if there is a suspicion of paroxysmal arrhythmias because a resting 12-lead ECG is unlikely to capture the event. Ambulatory ECGs can also be useful in considering heart rate variability, which may have an important prognostic value in heart failure (Panina et al. 1995). If occasional bursts of a potentially life-threatening arrhythmia, such as ventricular tachycardia, are seen then the patient with heart failure should be considered for an internal cardiac defibrillator (ICD). If there are periods of heart block then a pacemaker may be required. A 24-hour ECG can also help to guide drug therapy, for example, in the timing of medications to avoid bradycardia.

Unfortunately, if the symptom is very infrequent – perhaps the patient has palpitations once a month or so – the chances of this device capturing the event are small and an alternative such as an implantable internal loop recorder or patient activated monitor may be needed (Ng et al. 2004).

EXERCISE TOLERANCE TEST (ETT)

The Exercise Tolerance Test is a continuous 12-lead ECG recording carried out while the patient is put through staged exercise (usually either on a walking treadmill or bicycle). The test lasts for a maximum of 15 minutes and is carried out to a set standard protocol.

The purpose of the test is to increase cardiac oxygen demands. As the demand for oxygenated blood rises, supply must be increased. This involves raising the cardiac output through increases in heart rate and stroke volume. If supply fails to match demand then the myocardium will become ischaemic and changes such as ST segment depression or T wave inversion will be seen on the ECG recording. Provoking ischaemia is an indication there may be problems with the coronary arteries. An ischaemic patient may also have symptoms such as angina or breathlessness. There may also be haemodynamic abnormalities, such as a sudden drop in blood pressure, indicating a problem with blood flow from the heart.

The exercise tolerance test is an important way to investigate patients with suspected or known coronary artery disease. As the majority of patients with heart failure have a background of ischaemic heart disease, many will undergo this test. The test is also a useful method of assessing the functional capacity of someone with known heart failure. This if especially helpful if the patient is being assessed prior to an exercise training programme.

For a patient with severe heart failure, or with physical or mental incapacities, an exercise tolerance test may not be possible to perform safely. Sometimes patients may not be able to walk on a treadmill but could do a bicycle test. An alternative is to test the patient on a six-minute walk test (Kervio et al. 2004).

Patients with heart failure will usually have a low exercise tolerance and they are likely to become breathless early in the test. This has led to concerns that undertaking an exercise tolerance test may be harmful for these patients. There is no evidence that patients with heart failure are more likely to have complications during an exercise test than other patients. However, if the patient is unable to complete more than a minute or so of the test then only very limited data will be gained, so it may not be worth it.

ECHOCARDIOGRAM

The echocardiogram, or ultrasound imaging of the heart, is the current gold standard investigation for heart failure. It can provide great detail about the function and structure of the heart. Crucially, it is an investigation in real time, so any abnormalities in the movement or contractility of the heart can be seen. As well as the size and shape of the heart chambers, valves and myocardium, it is possible using Doppler techniques to assess the flow of blood through the heart. Intracardiac thrombi, occurring after myocardial infarction or if the patient has a clotting disorder or is in an irregular rhythm, can be detected by an echocardiogram. The functioning of the heart can be assessed and there are various ways of expressing abnormal dysfunction – perhaps the most widely known is the left ventricular ejection fraction (LVEF). Wall motion abnormalities and low ejection fractions are associated with poorer prognoses (Madsen et al. 1996; Solomon et al. 2005).

The echocardiogram is a relatively inexpensive investigation. There is an initial capital cost of purchasing the scanners (about £20 000–30 000 per machine) along with ongoing costs in maintenance, staff training and salaries. Traditionally, almost all echocardiogram services have been hospital based and it would be fair to say demand for the service outstripped supply in most hospitals in the past. As a result some areas have at times had long waiting times for outpatient echocardiograms. This was clearly unacceptable when it is the definitive diagnostic test for such a serious condition as heart failure (Davie & McMurray 1997). In recent years a lot of extra resources have been put in place and professionals have worked together on ways to use those resources most effectively – such as in open access echocardiogram heart failure services – with great improvement in accessibility to these services (Department of Health 2003).

Apart from hospitals providing echocardiograms there are alternative service models, for instance, buying scanning services from private providers or setting up community services (Partridge 2004). Any professional can be trained to carry out scans and some GPs and nurses have done so as part of primary care diagnostic developments for heart failure (Fox 2004). The British Society of Echocardiography (BSE) training and certification process assures echocardiography competency (Chambers et al. 2004). There has been some controversy over whether community-delivered scans are of a quality similar to those offered in hospital (Partridge 2004).

From a patient's perspective, having an echocardiogram is rarely unpleasant. The procedure involves a little jelly on the chest wall and some pressing with a probe. Occasionally patients can find the probe pressure a discomfort. The test itself usually only takes around a quarter to half an hour. In some centres that run a one-stop heart failure clinic, the results will be immediately available to the patient but in other areas the results will go to a senior doctor for reporting and this may lead to a delay.

Echocardiograms do have practical and clinical limitations. They are carried out and interpreted by human beings so there is some margin of error and variation between scans. It is not always possible to get good quality pictures from every patient, especially obese patients and those with lung diseases. Although echocardiograms are very good at detecting systolic dysfunction they are less effective in looking for diastolic dysfunction. Diastolic dysfunction is thought to be more widespread than previously thought but it is difficult to assess because the left ventricle stiffens with age and the point at which this becomes diastolic dysfunction is difficult to say. One method of looking for diastolic dysfunction is to measure the pattern of diastolic filling looking at early ('E' wave) and late ('A' wave) flow across the mitral valve using Doppler. Some measure of this can be seen if there is EA reversal, although EA reversal is also common with increased age.

The standard echocardiogram involves a transthoracic approach (TTE). An alternative is to get the patient to swallow a special probe to carry out a transoesophageal echocardiogram (TOE). The advantage of this method is that the image quality may be better as the probe is nearer to the heart without the chest wall and lung tissue being in the way. A transoesophageal echocardiogram is best for confirming an intracardiac thrombus and for looking in detail at the mitral valve. However, it is a more difficult procedure, involving more staff and the use of sedation. For the patient it is often very uncomfortable, although the use of amnesiac sedatives, such as midozolam, reduces the discomfort somewhat.

As well as helping to make a diagnosis, an echocardiogram is useful if the patient's condition changes. It is sometimes requested as a method of routinely assessing progress, for example in patients with genetic cardiomyopathy or a prosthetic cardiac valve. However, there is a question of whether all heart failure patients should receive routine scans. At one extreme it could be argued that they should be scanned only if the clinical situation changes or a significant change to treatment is planned. An alternative argument would be that a scan at regular intervals could assess progress. Although scanning does not, as far as we know, carry any direct risks to the patient, frequent scanning has implications, as mentioned earlier: there is an economic cost, an increase in waiting times and potentially an increase in anxiety for the patient. On the other hand, periodic scanning can reduce anxiety in some patients and enables changes to be picked up early in order to influence treatment decisions.

Another use of this investigative tool in heart failure is to carry out stress echocardiograms – usually using low dose dobutamine – to look for myocardial ischaemia. This is an alternative if the patient is unable to undertake an exercise tolerance test or if the results of an exercise test are inconclusive. The particular value of a stress echocardiogram is that it assesses whether there is any reversible ischaemia – indicating salvageable myocardium – when a patient is being considered for coronary revascularisation.

Box 7.5 Echocardiogram Findings in Heart Failure

Structure

- muscle hypertrophy
- chamber dilation
- aneurysms
- thrombi
- valve disease

Function

- wall motion abnormalities (dyskinesia, akinesia)
- dyssynchronicity
- reduced contractility
- reduced left ventricular function
- diastolic dysfunction

CHEST X-RAY (CXR)

A chest X-ray is usually recommended in guidelines as part of diagnostic testing for heart failure. It is also a frequent investigation in emergency departments if patients attend with suspected acute heart failure. As an investigation to confirm heart failure it has limitations but as most patients are being considered for heart failure as a result of breathlessness it is important to consider differential lung diagnoses – such as pleural effusions, pneumonia, emphysema, tuberculosis, tumours and fibrosis – which are aided by a chest X-ray.

In patients with heart failure the chest X-ray may show an enlarged heart, known as *cardiomegaly*. This may be as a result of dilation, hypertrophy or pericardial effusion. The cardiothoracic ratio, or the proportion of space between each side of the lungs at the widest point occupied by the heart, will be greater than 50 %. However, there are difficulties with interpreting whether some films do show enlargement and there can be a poor match between cardiothoracic ratio and left ventricular dysfunction (Clark & Coats 2000). Also, many patients will have heart failure without cardiac enlargement. As a result, the chest X-ray does not correlate well with echocardiograms in diagnosing heart failure.

There are other elements that the chest X-ray may reveal in patients with heart failure. It may pick up features suggestive of pulmonary oedema, such as congestion of the upper lobes, fluid in the horizontal fissures and Kerley B lines in the costrophrenic angles. Pulmonary oedema is usually only present in acute left ventricular failure. If pulmonary oedema is present, a provoking cause for acute left ventricular failure – such as a paroxysmal arrhythmia or myocardial infarction – needs urgent investigation, as well as treatment to stabilise the heart failure and remove the excess fluid. In severe cases of acute heart failure pleural effusions may also be present and visible on chest X-rays. This is not in or of itself diagnostic of heart failure as effusions are also caused by respiratory conditions such as lung cancer, pneumonia or pulmonary infarctions.

As well as clinical limitations, chest X-rays have practical limitations as an investigative method. Rarely are they available outside of hospital so requesting an X-ray means the patient will have to attend hospital. Although the procedure is usually quick and straightforward for the patient, the use of X-rays must be limited to the minimum needed for clinical practice because of the exposure to radiation.

BLOOD TESTS

Blood tests can aid in the diagnosis of heart failure and can provide valuable prognostic data by indicating if organs are well perfused. Having blood tests at regular intervals is an essential part of the follow-up of patients with heart failure in order to detect complications early on and to adjust treatment. The frequency of blood tests should be determined by the clinical situation.

BRAIN NATRIURETIC PEPTIDE (BNP)

There has been much interest in blood tests to measure for brain natriuretic peptide (BNP) in patients with heart failure. BNP was discovered in 1988 and is a stress enzyme released by the heart in response to high blood volume or wall pressure. BNP suppresses the renin-angiotensin-aldosterone system and acts as a vasodilator. When the heart is stressed BNP is released and patients with heart failure have a baseline abnormally high level – which is useful for diagnosis – that increases the more stress the heart is under. This is useful for prognosis (Cowie et al. 1997).

Studies of BNP agree that it has an excellent negative predictive value in heart failure. That is, a normal BNP level makes heart failure in an untreated patient unlikely. However, an abnormal BNP level is not necessarily due to heart failure. In other words, the positive predictive value is lower, so a patient with a positive BNP will need to have an echocardiogram to confirm or refute the diagnosis.

This pattern of good negative predictive value and poorer positive predictive value for BNP is almost identical to that of the ECG and used in a similar manner. The current NICE guidelines for chronic heart failure recommend that an ECG or BNP can be used as the initial investigation, with a positive test result triggering referral for an echocardiogram.

There has been some debate about whether a BNP test offers anything additional to an ECG. This is relevant because the cost of a BNP test is higher than an ECG – a BNP test currently costs around £10–15 an assay – although this cost is likely to fall if the test was used more widely. It is also highly probable that patients would still require an ECG as it provides a richness of data that a BNP test cannot.

A systematic review of comparisons of the diagnostic accuracy of ECGs, BNP tests and NT-pro BNP tests located 32 such studies. These showed that all three tests had similar sensitivity (> 80 %) and similar poor specificity. Combining ECGs and BNP tests did not improve sensitivity and there was limited evidence it might improve specificity. The review concludes that at the present time there is no evidence to justify the use of ECGs and BNP tests together and no evidence to justify the additional costs of BNP tests over ECGs (Davenport et al. 2006).

Like all tests the diagnostic accuracy of BNP tests depends on where the normal parameters are set – setting the normal level low means that a few patients with heart failure are likely to be missed but more people with abnormal results do not have heart failure (false positives); conversely, setting the normal level high means that fewer people without heart failure will get a positive result but some people with heart failure might get negative results (false negatives). As BNP in heart failure is relatively new, the issue of what is normal for the test is still being resolved (Latour-Perez et al. 2005).

Leaving aside their diagnostic use, there is increasing evidence that BNP tests may have a particular use in routine monitoring of the progress of the disease, especially looking for deterioration, and as a prognostic marker (Masson et al. 2006). A systematic review of 19 studies of the ability of BNP to act as a prognostic marker found that it was a strong indicator of risk the higher it was raised in patients with confirmed heart failure (Doust et al. 2005).

ELECTROLYTES AND RENAL FUNCTION

Renal dysfunction and heart failure often coexist. This is partly because both conditions are common but also because a poorly functioning heart does not perfuse the organs fully. Chapter 5 outlined the hormonal and haemodynamic interactions between the heart and kidneys. Many of the drugs used to treat heart failure, such as diuretics and ACE-inhibitors, also have an effect on the renal system. Some of the medication can disturb electrolyte balance, which is important for the electrical stability of the heart. Rapidly worsening renal function may require adjustments to heart failure treatment and is a marker of poor prognosis.

Urea and creatinine are by-products of metabolism that are excreted by the kidneys. If their levels are raised then it is a sign that the kidneys are not working well. Unfortunately, the tests for urea and creatinine levels, as a measure of renal function, have shortcomings and other more sensitive tests, such as estimated glomerular filtration rate (eGFR), are becoming more widely used. The serum levels of the electrolytes sodium and potassium, which are essential for the electrical stability of cells, are also checked routinely, along with urea and creatinine.

As a minimum, recommendation 62 of the NICE guidelines advises stable heart failure patients to have routine renal function tests every six months (NICE 2003). An unstable patient will require much more frequent monitoring, perhaps as often as daily in a hospitalised patient, to measure treatment effects. When changing medications that have renal effects, such as diuretics, ACE-inhibitors and aldosterone antagonists, close monitoring of renal function is necessary.

Interpreting the significance of abnormal results can be difficult. Patients with renal dysfunction may need referral to renal physicians and some areas have protocols based on eGFR levels to trigger these referrals. The average heart failure patient is elderly and renal function deteriorates naturally with age. By the time urea and creatinine are raised there may already be significant renal damage. There is also the difficult question as to what level of renal dysfunction is acceptable when ACE-inhibitors are started. The NICE guidelines for chronic heart failure advise that a baseline creatinine rise of up to 50 % or an absolute figure of up to 300 are acceptable but above this action is needed – a staged response of, firstly, reducing diuretics or vasodilators, then reducing the dose of ACE-inhibitor, and then referring to renal physicians if no improvement is advised.

There are also issues with regard to interpreting electrolyte test results. Low serum sodium levels, or hyponatraemia, occur in severe heart failure and are a poor prognostic indicator (Gheorghiade et al. 2007). It is not certain whether trying to increase the sodium level through medications is beneficial. It is worth noting that low sodium levels also occur in other conditions and these should be considered as differential causes.

High and low serum potassium levels, or hyperkaleamia and hypokaleamia, can cause arrhythmias. Both are seen in patients with heart failure. Hypokaleamia is usually caused by excessive diuresis. Levels can be raised using drugs such as slow-K or sando-K but care must be taken that these prescriptions are reviewed and stopped as soon as they are no longer needed. Hyperkaleamia in patients with heart failure usually occurs if the patient is taking an ACE-inhibitor, aldosterone antagonist or a potassium sparing diuretic. Hyperkaleamia is a particular concern in the elderly. An analysis of hospital admissions in Canada before and after the RALES trial showed that the use of spironolactone decreased heart failure admissions but increased hyperkalaemic admissions and death (Juurlink et al. 2004). The NICE guidelines recommend that a serum potassium level of up to 5.5 mmol/l is acceptable but beyond that there should be interventions to reduce the level by halving the dose. A potassium level of greater than 6.0 mmol/l should lead to the suspension of spironolactone (NICE 2003).

FULL BLOOD COUNT (FBC)

Patients with heart failure should have a full blood count at least once every six months. This is because of the high incidence of chronic anaemia in these patients. If haemoglobin and haematocrit levels are low then further blood tests – ferritin, folate and vitamin B12 levels – will be needed to diagnose the type of anaemia present. As most patients will be on blood thinning drugs and anti-platelet drugs, there is also a heightened risk of acute anaemia as a result of bleeding and full blood counts will be needed in any patient who has signs or symptoms of blood loss.

Haemoglobin, attached to red blood cells, carries oxygen around the body. So it is not surprising that anaemia can cause symptoms of fatigue and breathlessness. Vigilance is needed with patients with heart failure because they may well already have these symptoms chronically. Severe untreated anaemia can precipitate acute left ventricular failure.

Conversely, heart failure can be caused by the pressure of an over-production of iron. This is a condition called haemochromatosis and is a genetic disease that is thought to be under-diagnosed. Iron studies may reveal the presence of high ferritin levels and specialist referral would then be indicated.

A full blood count is also essential if there is concern that the patient may have an infection. Heart failure patients who get infections tend to become more ill than other people might and earlier diagnosis and treatment of infections is important. A full blood count of a patient with an infection may show elevated white blood cells. Other inflammatory markers, such as CRP and ESR, should also be requested at the same time in these circumstances.

LIVER FUNCTION TESTS (LFTS)

The liver is a major organ and uses a significant part of the cardiac output. Patients with chronic poor cardiac output can have this reflected in a reduction of liver function. Liver function tests are useful to consider cardiac function indirectly. However, most deranged liver function is not due to cardiac dysfunction and liver function tests are not a diagnostic test for heart failure. Liver function tests contain various assays and certain patterns of abnormalities point to different disorders.

Abnormal liver function tests may highlight potential aetiology of heart failure. Patients who are drinking to excess will tend to have an elevated gamma glutamyl traspeptidase (GGT) – although again, not every patient with a raised GGT is a drinker.

Periodic checking of liver function is also necessary if the patient is taking certain cardiac medication or if the patient is taking the medication and feels unwell. Drugs such as amiodarone and statins, both widely used in patients with heart failure, can provoke liver dysfunction.

THYROID FUNCTION TESTS (TFTS)

An overactive thyroid gland can lead to tachycardia, which can in turn lead to acute left ventricular failure. If there are no underlying structural problems with the heart then thyrotoxicosis is a reversible cause of heart failure. Equally possible, however, is the situation where an overactive thyroid leads to acute left ventricular failure because the patient has an unconnected background of chronic heart failure. In other words, asymptomatic chronic heart failure has been unmasked by an acute event.

Checking thyroid function is important in any patient complaining of palpitations, agitation or excessive fatigue.

The second circumstance in which patients with heart failure will need thyroid function tests is if they are taking amiodarone. This drug contains iodine and can cause hypothyroidism or hyperthyroidism. Patients taking amiodarone should have thyroid function tests at least every six months (NICE 2003).

CHOLESTEROL AND GLUCOSE

Although there is not a clear link between heart failure and high cholesterol levels there is a strong indirect link, in that high cholesterol is a major risk factor for ischaemic heart disease and the majority of patients with heart failure have ischaemic heart disease. Cholesterol testing should be part of any initial screening and regular follow-up.

Diabetes is believed to cause a particular cardiomyopathy in some patients. The link between diabetes and ischaemic heart disease is very strong. For this reason it is important to investigate whether the patient may have diabetes, if this has not already been done. If they are diabetic then there is evidence from the United Kingdom Prospective Diabetes Study that the tightness of the control of the blood sugars affects cardiac outcomes (The UKPDS Group 1998).

Generally, regular cholesterol and glucose checks will be arranged in primary care as part of annual cardiovascular disease clinics and population screening in older patients.

Box 7.6 Adult Blood Test Normal Ranges

Test	Lower range	Upper range
BNP	< 50 pmol/l is seen as normal	> 150 pmol/l is suspicious of heart failure
Sodium	133 mmol/l	148 mmol/l
Potassium	3.5 mmol/l	5.5 mmol/l
Urea	1.7 mmol/l	8.3 mmol/l
Creatinine	Male 73 μmol/l	Male 126 μmol/l
	Female 44 μmol/l	Female 80 μmol/l
eGFR	90 +	Normal
	60–89	Mild renal dysfunction
	30–59	Moderate renal dysfunction
	15–29	Severe renal dysfunction
	< 15	End stage renal dysfunction
Haemoglobin	Male 13.5 g/dl	Male 18.0 g/dl
	Female 11.5 g/dl	Female 16.0 g/dl
WBC	4.0 (10^9/l)	11.0 (10^9/l)

CARDIAC CATHETERISATION

Patients with heart failure may need cardiac catheterisation. This is the directing of a fine bore tube through the blood vessels back to the heart. This can be through the venous system back to the vena cava, right atrium, right ventricle and pulmonary artery, or through the arterial system back to the aorta, coronary arteries and left ventricle.

Although cardiac catheterisation is a technique pioneered by doctors, nurses are involved in several ways: preparing the patients, assisting during the procedure and in recovery afterwards. Additionally, there are developments whereby additional trained advanced practitioners are now performing angiographies.

RIGHT HEART CATHETERISATION

The first right heart catheterisation was carried out in 1929 by a German doctor just out of training, Werner Forssmann, on himself (Meyer 1990). The technique is used in cardiac catheter laboratories as part of electrophysiology procedures and in coronary care units and intensive care units as part of the haemodynamic monitoring of acutely unwell patients. For haemodynamic monitoring, a pulmonary artery catheter (also known as Swan Ganz after two early pioneers) is inserted percutaneously through a central vein to the right side of the heart and then to the pulmonary artery. It enables a range of haemodynamic measures to be calculated including central venous pressure (CVP) or right atrial pressure (RAP), right ventricular pressure (RVP), pulmonary artery pressure (PAP), pulmonary artery capillary wedge pressure (PACWP) and cardiac output (CO). This data can be useful in diagnosing and guiding treatment of acutely unwell patients in heart failure.

There are several disadvantages of pulmonary artery catheterisation. It is only available to a minority of seriously ill, hospitalised heart failure patients. This is unlikely to change as it remains costly in terms of equipment and staff training. Having a line inserted into the heart from the skin is a serious potential infection risk and the catheter should be removed as soon as possible. The most important criticism of pulmonary artery catheters is that in practice the measurements often lack accuracy and their accuracy is too dependent on additional variables such as operator skill. It would be fair to say that right-sided heart catheterisation, outside of cardiac catheter laboratories, has declined in use since being pioneered in the 1970s.

LEFT HEART CATHETERISATION

The most common indication for left-sided heart catheterisation is coronary angiography. In this technique a radioisotope is injected into the coronary vessels and filmed using X-rays to outline features. For heart failure patients, a coronary angiogram will help to confirm the cause of their condition – ischaemic or non-ischaemic – by identifying coronary lesions and areas of poor myocardial perfusion.

Left side catheterisation can also provide further information if the aortic valve is passed. The gradient of any aortic stenosis can be calculated. The shape of the left ventricle can be outlined and the left ventricular ejection fraction calculated.

Left-sided cardiac catheterisation is now a common procedure and is very safe for the majority of patients. It does, however, come with risks, both minor and serious, which sadly lead to some rare fatalities.

IMPEDANCE CARDIOGRAPHY (ICG)

Impedance cardiography uses four double electrodes to send a small electrical signal through the body and measure the electrical differences at the same time as recording the patient's ECG. As different mediums conduct electricity differently it is possible to measure the aortic waveform and plot this against the ECG. This allows various haemodynamic measurements such as stroke volume (SV), cardiac output (CO) and cardiac index (CI), as well as indicating thoracic fluid content (TFC) and measuring the timing of different aspects of the cardiac cycle. An ICG can measure thoracic fluid volume because this is inversely proportional to mean thoracic electrical impedance (Zo) and it may be more sensitive in detecting pulmonary fluid than a chest X-ray (Peacock et al. 2000).

The technique was developed from technology used in the 1970s American space programme and has mainly been used in intensive care units in the United States. It has been trialled against measurements from right-sided heart catheterisation and found to be of equal accuracy. It has the clear advantage of being non-invasive and virtually risk-free.

There has been interest in using the equipment to evaluate patients with heart failure (Summers et al. 2006). The recent PREDICT study showed that a combination of parameters from the monitor was a strong predictor of outcomes in patients with heart failure (Packer et al. 2006). With the improvements in computerisation it is now possible to get a portable version that can be carried out to patients' homes. This enables more accurate monitoring of their condition and early detection of deterioration, and provides better data to justify adjustments to treatment rather than clinical assessment alone.

One of the biventricular defibrillators/internal defibrillators (*InSync Sentry*) has a measuring option for intrathoracic impedance with a built-in audible alarm as a warning sign of pulmonary fluid retention in heart failure patients (Ypenburg et al. 2007)

NUCLEAR IMAGING

Nuclear imaging can give useful information as to cardiac structure and function. There is a range of different investigations available but relatively few heart failure patients undergo these procedures. The procedures are technically complex and are done in larger hospitals and research centres.

Radionuclide ventriculography or multi-gated acquisition (MUGA) scans give a precise left ventricular ejection fraction and allow regional wall motion abnormalities to be seen. The scans tend to be of poorer quality in patients with abnormal cardiac rhythms. As the scan involves a dose of radiation it should be used cautiously and only where there is a clear clinical need.

Myocardial perfusion imaging usually allows visualisation of myocardial ischaemia. It is more accurate than exercise tolerance tests in finding ischaemia and is equivalent to stress echocardiograms. It is often requested to detect if there is any viable myocardium in patients who may be considered for revascularisation.

The number of magnetic resonance imaging (MRI) scanners and the uses they are put to has increased a great deal in recent years. There has been much interest in cardiac applications for MRI scanners as they are especially useful in allowing accurate assessments of body structures. The latest generation of scanners allows real-time scanning of cardiac volumes, muscle mass, contractility, tissue scarring and cardiac function and can give a very accurate left ventricular ejection fraction measurement (Azevedo et al. 2005). Another use for cardiac MRI is to assess the scope of myocardial ischaemia. Coronary angiography using MRI is practicable although this is currently generally limited to research projects rather than clinical use.

There are several practical drawbacks to more widespread use of cardiac MRI scanning at present: there are a limited number of scanners; they are not located conveniently for all patients; many other medical specialties wish to use the scanners; and there are a limited number of scanning time slots and consequent waiting times. It is likely that in the near future the extra information or accuracy gained from a cardiac MRI scan is going to be considered necessary – or have enough benefit over traditional techniques to justify the extra cost and inconvenience – in only a minority of heart failure patients.

Part III Treatment

8 Treatment Essentials

In this chapter the fundamentals of treatment are discussed. The importance of the education of patients and their carers about their condition is discussed and how this can be done. Specific information that should be given to all patients is outlined. The effects of lifestyle modifications on heart failure are explained. The psychological impact, including conditions such as anxiety and depression, on patients is considered. Strategies for achieving patient concordance and self-management are introduced. The roles of specialist allied healthcare professionals, support associations and social services are outlined.

Box 8.1 Summary of Non-Pharmacological Treatments

Education	• about the condition
	• self-monitoring
Information	• travel
	• driving
	• sexual relations
	• immunisation
	• welfare rights
	• support groups
Lifestyle	• exercise
	• diet, water and salt
	• smoking and alcohol
	• sleeping
	• stress

EDUCATION

A newly-diagnosed patient will have several questions in mind – *What is heart failure? How did I get it? Can it be cured? How will it be treated? What does it mean to my life and my future?* Patients often need a little time to ask these questions and the questions may come up repeatedly as the patient comes to terms with their condition. Patients need to have explanations that make sense to them and that are not overly technical or unduly complex. Many patients misunderstand what heart failure means and a majority of them are poorly informed about their condition. It is known that patients who understand their condition and why their treatment is important are more likely to be concordant with that treatment and thereby have fewer complications and better outcomes (C. Anderson et al. 2005; Gwadry-Sridhar et al. 2005).

There are a number of issues to explain and discuss with the patient about diagnosis, prognosis and the effects of their condition on them. It may be difficult to cover all of these in a short clinic appointment but information is also less likely to be retained by the patient if the consultation is too lengthy. It is probably advisable to split the information over a couple of consultations to reduce information overload and to allow the information to be understood. The use of written information can help to reinforce messages – the British Heart Foundation has an excellent series of patient information leaflets available (see Box 8.2). However, it is important not to rely on written information, as not all patients who take leaflets will actually read them. It can also be helpful to supply a contact number for the heart failure service so that the patient can phone to clarify any outstanding information.

Box 8.2 British Heart Foundation Publications Web Link

http://www.bhf.org.uk/publications.aspx

SELF-MANAGEMENT

Some heart failure patients, who are well educated about their condition, may be able to undertake a degree of self-management. In particular, they may be able to monitor their condition, detect early signs of fluid retention and adjust diuretic doses in response (Caldwell et al. 2005). This is helpful because the earlier that intervention is started to remove fluid retention, the less likely the patient is to become seriously ill and require hospitalisation (Jovicic et al. 2006). It meets the ethical ideal that all care should be a partnership between professionals, caregivers and the patient and gives the patient some control over the otherwise disempowering condition of heart failure (Flynn et al. 2005). Patients with heart failure, who feel they have less control, are more likely to suffer anxiety and depression (Joekes et al. 2007).

Not all patients will be able to participate actively in making decisions about their condition, for a variety of physical, psychological or psychiatric reasons. The degree to which patients can self-manage will depend on the patient, their level of understanding of their condition and the complexity of treatment.

Most patients will be able to participate in regular weighing to de. retention. Not all heart failure patients retain fluid and weighing is more impo. for some than others. Some patients should weigh themselves daily while others may get by with twice a week. They should watch out for a rapid weight increase, as this is more likely to be caused by fluid than solids. Precisely how much weight gain should be looked out for over and what time span is a little arbitrary – an easy-to-remember guide is 3 kg over a week for an average-sized man and 2 kg for an average-sized woman. If there is a sudden weight increase, this should trigger a heart failure review and probably a temporary adjustment of treatment, particularly changes to diuretics. If the patient understands their condition well enough they can be given a planned response to weight increase involving a temporary increase in diuretics, which they can commence. They should still of course be reviewed at the earliest opportunity.

Clinicians are often nervous about sanctioning patients adjusting after own medication. Certainly, it would not be advisable for patients themselves to start adjusting doses of ACE-inhibitors or beta-blockers. With diuretics, the reality is that many patients already miss or change doses for social reasons. Rather than turn a blind eye to this it seems more sensible to acknowledge the reasons patients do so and work with them to achieve concordance, even though this means ceding some decision-making power to those patients.

INFORMATION

Patients require specific information with regard to their heart failure and matters of travel, insurance, driving, welfare rights and support groups. Not all patients will need all this information or need it all at once. None the less, it can be a lot of information to go through in a consultation. Some of it can be given in written form – NICE and British Heart Foundation booklets are available – for the patient to take away and read in their own time. However, not all patients read well, or in English, and sometimes patients will forget to read information they have been given.

These barriers to giving patients information can be overcome in a few ways. As mentioned earlier, giving the patients a contact number so that they can get in touch if they have further questions is a useful additional strategy. It will need to be made clear to patients that the telephone is not manned all the time (unless a 24-hour service is available) and that a voicemail or answer machine service is set up on the line to avoid missed calls. If patients are seen regularly there will be an opportunity to provide information in smaller chunks and to check that information has been understood. It is also possible to give certain types of information mainly at the appropriate time of year: for example, holiday bookings are possibly more likely to be made in late winter or early spring, and immunisations take place in autumn.

with regard to travel for patients with heart failure. For
fit to travel, especially by air? Will they be able to get
happen if they become ill abroad?
, if a patient can climb a flight of stairs unaided then they are
ı. That said, stability needs to be considered and if a patient is in
ɔility or has evidence of fluid retention, it would be advisable not
to ⸴   ᴀought that unstable patients with fluid retention may be affected by
flying aᴠ   altitude because of the pressure changes and arterial hypoxia effect of
high altitude (Squires 1985). In fact, most patients with heart failure do fly without
any adverse effects. If there are concerns then sensible advice is to avoid long-haul
flights or split the journey with a stopover.

Travel insurance is a wise precaution for all travellers but especially so for
patients with heart failure. If someone is taken ill abroad the cost of treatment and
repatriation to the United Kingdom can be very high. The cost of travel insurance
will be higher than for a person before they had heart failure. This is not surprising,
as they are a higher insurance risk. Sometimes patients can struggle to find an
insurer but some companies do specialise in patients with medical problems and the
British Heart Foundation website contains some links to companies that will insure
patients with cardiac conditions. Patients should be reminded that not disclosing
their medical condition will invalidate any insurance they take out.

If travelling abroad patients will fall outside of the NHS. The United Kingdom
does, however, have reciprocal arrangements with many countries, especially in
Europe, to provide emergency healthcare. A list of countries with which the United
Kingdom has arrangements is listed in Box 8.3 and it is advised that patients

---

Box 8.3 Countries with Reciprocal Health Agreements with the UK

Reciprocal health agreements with UK	No reciprocal health agreements with UK
• Austria	• Turkey
• Belgium	• Canada
• Cyprus	• Turkey
• Czech Republic	• Canada
• Denmark	• United States and Mexico
• Estonia	• most Caribbean islands
• Finland	• South America
• France	• the Middle East
• Germany	• Africa
• Greece	• most of Asia (including India, Thailand,
• Hungary	Japan and Hong Kong)

Box 8.3 (Continued)

- Iceland
- Ireland
- Italy
- Latvia
- Liechtenstein
- Lithuania
- Luxembourg
- Malta
- The Netherlands
- Norway
- Poland
- Portugal
- Slovakia
- Slovenia
- Spain (including the Canary and Balearic Islands)
- Sweden
- Switzerland

- the whole Pacific region (except Australia and New Zealand)

check the Department of Health website to confirm these details and check for any changes before making their arrangements. The patient needs to collect a European Health Insurance Card (the replacement for the E111 form) which can be applied for online or from the Post Office. Patients may also want advice on medical facilities available at their destination. As a general rule, travel within the developed world will offer the same level of heart failure care as in the United Kingdom but patients might perhaps be more cautious about travel to more out of the way destinations. Also, hot and humid climates may make symptoms less tolerable.

Travel within the United Kingdom will rarely be a problem for patients with heart failure as the distances involved are relatively short. That said, all travel can be difficult socially for patients on diuretics. Some common sense is needed. Many patients can miss doses of diuretics without adverse effects. Diuretics could be taken earlier or later within the day – although after 4 pm may lead to a disturbed night's sleep – as although for many patients loop diuretics work in around half an hour they can continue to have an effect for up to six hours. For others, their instability will mean they cannot miss doses of diuretics but may be able to get by with a reduced dose for that day. Alternatively, adaptation of the journey will be needed either through planning more frequent stops or travelling by a method that enables bathroom facilities (such as the train or coach).

DRIVING

Driving is important in most people's lives and patients with heart failure are worried that they may be forced to stop driving. Heart failure, unlike myocardial infarctions, is not usually notifiable to the DVLA. There are a couple of exceptions to this general rule. The first is if the patient is having symptoms that may affect their driving – such as severe breathlessness at rest, syncope or fatigue leading to drowsiness. In these cases the DVLA should be informed and the patient should not drive. The second exception is that patients who drive with Public Vehicle Licences or Heavy Goods Vehicle Licences have to inform the DVLA of their medical condition and are not likely to be able to drive professionally again.

It is the patient's responsibility to inform the DVLA of any medical reasons why they may not be able to drive. Failure to do so is an offence and would also invalidate car insurance. If a clinician has a suspicion that a patient has not informed the DVLA of a notifiable condition then they have a duty to report the matter. Further details on the medical regulations relating to driving can be found on the DVLA website.

Box 8.4 Medical Guidelines on Driving

http://www.dvla.gov.uk/medical.aspx

SEXUAL RELATIONSHIPS

Patients and their partners are often concerned about how heart failure affects their sexual relationship. Sex is an important part of most people's lives but it is private and people do not usually like to talk about it and may feel inhibited in doing so. The same inhibitions are also likely to affect the clinician and this is an area where good communication skills are important to both broach the subject and deal with it successfully.

Heart failure affects sexual activity both directly and indirectly. Patients may have a loss of interest, find difficulty with arousal or have erectile dysfunction. The medications for heart failure are often a further cause of sexual dysfunction, especially erection difficulties, through lowering of the blood pressure and peripheral circulation. This is a well-known side-effect for patients taking beta-blockers but also occurs with ACE-inhibitors and other vasodilators. Heart failure can also reduce libido where there are chronic symptoms such as exertional breathlessness, fatigue, anxiety and depression.

Psychological issues are a significant cause of sexual dysfunction. In patients with heart failure, they or their partner may well be concerned that sex is too dangerous. There is an element of truth in this assumption as the more functionally severe the heart failure, the more likely decompensation may be triggered by sexual activity (DeBusk et al. 2000). This rather depends upon what sexual activity is being undertaken as some activities and positions are more vigorous than others. The psychological benefits of an active sex live must be placed against any small increased risk of decompensation.

If we think of sex as exercise then it may be that the cardiac benefits of exercise, as discussed in Chapter 9, also apply to sex. Having said that, it is important to consider the patient in front of you. When you are advising an exercise-training regime for a patient, you should set them parameters – broadly speaking, to start gently and gradually increase the level of the activity – the same principle applies to advising patients on their fitness for sex.

For patients with ongoing sexual dysfunction, a referral to a specialist may be indicated. Treatments include counselling, penile injections, medications and mechanical devices. There is still misunderstanding amongst some professionals and patients that drugs to stimulate erection – such as sildenafil (*Viagra®*) – are contra-indicated in cardiac patients. This is not the case; the contra-indication is if a patient is taking a long-acting nitrate or requiring frequent short-acting glyceryl trinitrate (GTN) as a result of angina.

A practical question that arises if the patient has persistent sexual dysfunction is whether the beta-blockers or vasodilators should be stopped. This is a difficult decision for several reasons. It may be that for that patient the sexual dysfunction has no direct link with the medication, and that psychological issues or depression may perhaps be the underlying cause. If the medication is stopped the patient will not receive the prognostic benefits of taking the drug. Stopping medications should only be done after all other avenues have been examined and treatments tried, and if the loss of sexual function is important to the patient.

IMMUNISATION

For patients with heart failure, any serious infection increases haemodynamic strain on the heart, putting them at risk of acute cardiac decompensation. The most common forms of serious infections in the elderly are chest infections. Fortunately, it is now possible to have immunisation against influenza and pneumonia. The influenza immunisation is given annually and the pneumonia immunisation provides cover for many years. Having the immunisations does not, of course, guarantee that the patient might not catch these infections, as there are numerous strains around and not all can be included in the injection. Immunisation is recommended for vulnerable groups and this includes patients with heart failure. As GP surgeries gain funding as a result of achieving immunisation targets, they have systems in place to reach the target populations. It is worth while to remind patients opportunistically of the value of immunisations to increase uptake rates.

WELFARE RIGHTS

Heart failure can make working difficult and can mean that patients need extra support to manage their daily lives. These facts might have financial implications for patients and their carers. Patients may be entitled to state benefits but the system is complex, with different government departments and agencies being responsible for different benefits and allowances. Claiming one benefit may influence entitlement to others. Getting the best outcome depends on individual assessment of circumstances. Fortunately, in most areas help is available through two sources – the Citizens Advice Bureaux and the local council's Welfare Rights advice services. Both of these are free to use and give independent advice.

There are two principal non-means-tested, non-contribution-based financial benefits: the Disability Living Allowance (DLA) and the Attendance Allowance. The DLA is for people younger than 65 years old and the Attendance Allowance is for people older than 65 years. The DLA has two components, mobility and a personal care element, with people being allocated different levels within these two elements. The DLA is generally unaffected by income and people can work and claim this allowance. It is by no means automatic that patients with heart failure will be entitled to the DLA. Getting an expert, such as an adviser from the Welfare Rights department, to check the form before sending it is sensible as patients often fill in information on the forms in such a way that it is more likely to be refused. There is a right of appeal if patients are initially rejected. If patients are terminally ill, which is defined as a reasonable expectation of death within six months in this context, the process of claiming the DLA can be speeded up and simplified. The Attendance Allowance is similar to the DLA except that it applies to people of state retirement age and has a care component only but no mobility component.

There are a number of other benefits that circumstances might make a patient or their family eligible for, such as the Carer's Allowance and Council Tax Reduction. It is difficult to keep abreast of all of these entitlements, which is why the help of benefits experts can be useful – see Box 8.5 for web links. One area of inequity is that patients with heart failure are not entitled to free prescriptions – in the way that people with diabetes, for example, are automatically entitled to them. This can be a considerable cost. Fortunately, most patients are entitled to free prescriptions by virtue of being older than 60 years of age. Some patients may be entitled to free prescriptions due to a low income. For the others, pre-payment of prescription costs is usually the most cost-effective method of covering the cost.

Box 8.5 Welfare Rights Organisations Web Links

Citizens Advice Bureaux
http://www.adviceguide.org.uk/
Government Central Online Help Desk
http://www.direct.gov.uk/en/index.htm

The Welfare Rights Departments are run by local authorities – see their individual websites for contact details.

SUPPORT GROUPS

Patients may wish to participate in support groups. Nationally, the main cardiac support group is the British Heart Foundation charity, which has local branches. There may already be existing local patient support groups or patients may wish to set up their own. Often existing groups will not be specific to heart failure patients and may be more orientated to patients who have had heart attacks or cardiac surgery. Patients sometimes prefer support that is not so condition-focused. Organisations such as Age Concern can be very helpful in providing support to patients and their families in a number of practical and psychological ways.

Box 8.6 National Patient and Carers Support Association Web Links

http://www.bhf.org.uk/
http://www.carersuk.org/Home
http://www.ageconcern.org.uk/

LIFESTYLE

It is clear that many patients with heart failure have a lifestyle that contributes to their ill-health – either through obesity, smoking, diabetes, high blood pressure, poor diet or alcohol-related problems. On an individual basis, it is very difficult to say how far lifestyle affects the condition as there are too many complex variables. Indeed, some patients may have a completely healthy lifestyle and still develop heart failure. Other patients may have had risk factors, such as hypertension, for many years without being aware of it. It is best to avoid concepts such as blame when discussing lifestyle but important to explain how improving lifestyle affects quality of life, symptoms, complications and prognosis.

Making changes to a healthier lifestyle is an important element in treatment. An individualised assessment is needed to establish where changes in lifestyle may be important for the individual patient. Research suggests patients often believe they are following healthy lifestyle advice yet when objectively recorded their lifestyle is less healthy than reported (Sneed & Paul 2003). A degree of risk analysis needs to take place – for example, an alcoholic with heart failure and who continues to drink is not going to survive long. If the same patient has high cholesterol this is less of a priority than stopping drinking, although ideally patients will address all their lifestyle issues. In reality, for some patients it is psychologically overwhelming to try to make a lot of changes at once, so it is often better to prioritise and plan changes consecutively. For others, a heart failure diagnosis can act as a defining moment to spur them on to a new beginning.

Lifestyle change is difficult and many patients are sceptical as to whether it will make a difference. This is difficult to judge as some changes will be prophylactic in that they are to avoid problems – such as cholesterol reduction – but will not necessarily know what difference it has made in their case. There are other changes, such as reducing obesity and increasing exercise, which will improve functional status and have benefits that are visible. Most lifestyle changes will have benefits in the medium to long term; expecting sudden improvements in the short term is unrealistic. It is also worth remembering that the patient's condition may deteriorate, in the same period they are improving their lifestyle, for other reasons – and this can strain their commitment to continue.

Personality, beliefs and psychology are important elements in successful change to a healthier lifestyle. People are generally reasonably informed and it is not simple ignorance of the facts that leads to them continuing unhealthy practices. For example, after years of public health campaigns everyone knows smoking is bad for them but many continue, even after cardiac events or after respiratory complications begin. Their reasons as to why they continue may be complex – perhaps they enjoy smoking, perhaps it is part of their social or domestic circumstances, or they may feel addicted – all of which are psychological barriers to change that are individual to the patient. In order to assist the patient to live a healthier lifestyle, it is not enough merely to tell them their lifestyle is unhealthy. It is necessary to individualise the problem for them, to understand their perspective, to ascertain if they want to change and if so, to provide assistance and options for doing so, as well as to support, encourage and act as a resource for extra help.

EXERCISE

It used to be thought that patients with heart failure should 'rest' their hearts and avoid exercise. This is completely the opposite to current thinking, which is that patients with heart failure need to exercise to improve both their symptoms and their prognosis. This is such an important part of treatment that it will be discussed in depth in a separate chapter (Chapter 9).

DIET

Heart failure affects, and can be affected by, diet in a number of ways. Some people believe that diet has a more central role than previously thought and there are certainly many aspects of how diet affects the heart that are not yet fully understood. There are some general principles that can be applied but advice needs to be individualised to take into account patients' co-morbidities, such as renal failure or diabetes. There is no off-the-peg heart failure diet that all patients can follow.

Two thirds of patients with heart failure have ischaemic heart disease. These patients should be advised on reducing their cholesterol, as high cholesterol is a risk factor for cardiovascular disease. The laboratory definition of high cholesterol has fallen over the years, as more has been understood about the cardiac effects of higher cholesterol levels. The average total cholesterol in the United Kingdom is 5.2 mmol/l but the target for patients with heart disease is less than 4 mmol/l.

For patients with high cholesterol a low cholesterol diet should be advised – that is, low in dairy products, eggs and red meat. In a clinical trial that took place using the strict food controls of a prison, the best total cholesterol reduction with diet alone was 15 %. This means that, for most people with high cholesterol, medication will be necessary to achieve target levels. Fortunately, the statin drug group has been shown in extensive clinical trials to have the ability to reduce cholesterol by around a third.

Patients with diabetes mellitus and heart failure should be encouraged to keep their blood sugar under control. There is a clear link between uncontrolled diabetes and a range of complications, including cardiovascular complications.

Patients with heart failure frequently have chronic anaemia. This also tends to occur with patients with renal disease and the two may be linked. If anaemia occurs it can worsen symptoms of breathlessness and fatigue as well as making the heart work harder to compensate for the smaller amount of oxygenated blood being circulated. Sometimes changes in diet can correct or at least help to address problems of anaemia by adding more iron rich foods, such as fresh green vegetables.

It is important also to be aware of cultural differences in diet. For example, in Asian cultures food is strongly bound with love and respect. When people are sick they are offered rich, festival food to show how valued they are. The food may not be what a clinician would advise, often being high in fats and sugars, but its positive, immediate psychological value may outweigh the long-term negative nutritional aspects. Trying to remove the food in question may create family tension and psychological distress.

OBESITY

Analysis from the Framingham study has shown that obesity is a risk factor for the development of heart failure (Kenchaiah et al. 2002). This is as an independent risk factor and not only as a result of the links between obesity, hypertension and diabetes.

There may well be several mechanisms by which obesity contributes to heart failure. A severely overweight patient may develop haemodynamic changes such as volume overload, with increases in afterload and preload, left ventricular hyper-trophy, left ventricular dilation and remodelling (Lauer et al. 1991). In simple terms, if a patient is overweight then their heart will have to work harder all the time. There are also metabolic changes that affect the development of heart failure and obesity may be involved in these processes.

Distribution of fat appears to be at least as important as overall weight or body mass index (BMI). Abdominal obesity is now known to be associated with higher cardiovascular and heart failure risk (Rexrode et al. 1998; Lakka et al. 2002; Nicklas et al. 2006). This can be measured easily by waist size and waist-to-hip ratio.

Although obesity is a risk factor for heart failure there is a paradox in obese patients who already have heart failure: in many studies, overweight patients with heart failure have had better outcomes than those with lower body mass indexes

(Bozkurt & Deswal. 2005; Hall et al. 2005; Curtis et al. 2005). Why this apparently illogical phenomenon should exist is unknown. There are various theories linked to inflammation, metabolism and to the better ability of obese patients to tolerate higher doses of cardiac drugs (Hall et al. 2005). It is perhaps worth noting in this context that body mass index is a crude measure as it takes no account of fitness (muscle being heavier than fat) or of fat distribution.

Expert consensus is that despite this paradox, obese heart failure patients should be helped to reduce their weight. Obesity can sometimes provoke symptoms – such as orthopnoea, peripheral oedema, exertional dyspnoea, fatigue and sleep apnoea – which mimic heart failure (Massie 2002). The symptoms of heart failure are worsened by obesity and reducing obesity does have a positive effect on symptoms and NYHA functional heart failure class (Mariotti et al. 2004).

Losing excess weight is of course easier to say than to do. The first step is to make sure the patient understands why weight control is important for heart failure. Discussing weight needs sensitivity – obese patients are aware they are overweight but may be defensive and self-justifying about their weight because society views obesity negatively. Clinicians should be clear and practical and avoid value judgements.

Patients need to understand the mechanisms of weight gain. For most people it is a simple mechanism of energy in versus energy out, with the balance being stored as excess weight, influenced by hereditary factors and co-morbidities. For most patients with heart failure the change over time has been that they are using less energy as they are doing less, in response to symptoms. It is useful to have a plan and to set targets for weight loss. Be careful not to be too ambitious. It is sensible to agree staged aims for weight reduction. How this is done will depend upon the psychology of the patient. Crash diets are to be avoided. It is important to emphasise to the patient that in most commercial diets the initial impressive weight loss is of fluid and the patient is unlikely to achieve this because they are already on diuretics. Most patients will be able to increase the amount of energy they use through exercise. Many of the patients may not feel they are eating too much. This may be true or it may not – some people underestimate their intake unconsciously – and filling in a food chart can be useful to help these people recognise they are eating too much. Other people tell professionals what they want to hear to avoid confronting the situation. These people need to have the long-term effects of obesity on heart failure explained clearly. If they then choose not to address the issue then, ultimately, that is their choice as an adult and the patient should continue to be respected even if the professional does not condone the decision. The door must also be left open for change in the future.

For some patients referral to a dietitian can be helpful. This can also be a useful mechanism psychologically to restimulate the patient's commitment to try to lose weight. Formal programmes for weight control exist in some areas and may include nutritional counselling, physical activity, drug interventions, possible surgery, motivational support and lifestyle modification (Evangelista & Miller 2006). There are numerous examples of successful programmes that can be used as templates for people setting up weight loss programmes (Coviello & Nystrom 2003).

CARDIAC CACHEXIA

Some patients with advanced heart failure may develop cardiac cachexia, which carries a poor prognosis (Davos et al. 2003). Cachexia is evident in loss of skeletal muscle bulk. The loss of muscle means that some symptoms, especially fatigue and breathlessness, are likely to worsen. The cause of the cachexia is not fully understood but it is likely to be a result of a combination of poor appetite, poor absorption and abnormal metabolism, all resulting from poor perfusion of the gastro-intestinal tract in severe heart failure. These patients need expert advice and should be referred to a dietitian.

WATER AND SALT

Patients with heart failure are sometimes advised to restrict the amount of fluid they drink. The rationale is that the more fluid taken in the greater the risk of fluid retention. Although superficially logical this may be too simplistic physiologically, as the body will attempt to counterbalance any changes in fluid intake by reducing or increasing diuresis. As most patients will be on diuretics, restricting fluid may well be unnecessary, while also increasing the risk of dehydration and confusion – especially in the elderly. Fluid restrictions are never popular with patients and concordance is poor.

Whilst routinely advising fluid restrictions is not recommended, there are a few circumstances where it may be considered. If a patient is admitted to hospital with acute fluid retention then traditionally they will have a fluid restriction imposed – yet whether this is necessary is debatable and there is no strong evidence to support the practice (NICE 2003). Occasionally, patients may drink excessive volumes of fluid, usually in the mistaken belief it will be of benefit to their health. A normal fluid intake in an adult would be 3 or 4 litres a day and drinking a lot more than this may provoke decompensation due to volume overload in patients with heart failure. Some renal patients are advised to have oral fluid restrictions if on renal dialysis.

Restriction in dietary salt is also often advised for patients with heart failure. This is because physiologically water follows salt by osmosis in the body. Patients with heart failure may also have renal disease and may be less able to excrete salt; a high salt intake can result in fluid retention and increased end diastolic and systolic pressures (Volpe et al. 1993). Reduction in dietary salt can improve symptoms and haemodynamic function (Cody et al. 1994). Reducing salt increases the effectiveness of diuretics. In addition, as we saw in Chapter 5, heart failure patients are at risk of the hormonal triggering of salt and water retention, as a response to declining cardiac output. Non-adherence to low salt recommendations has been suggested to be responsible for a high proportion of heart failure admissions (Moser et al. 2004). For these reasons patients are advised to limit or reduce their salt intake.

As a general rule, most diets contain more than enough salt for the body's needs (2–3 g per day) but most people actually ingest a lot more because salt is hidden in processed foods, as a preservative and flavour enhancer, or because the patient adds salt to their food during cooking or at the table.

Traditionally, patients with heart failure often did not receive an assessment of their salt intake, nor any specific recommendations. Patients should be advised to switch to non-processed foods, which will also contain more vitamins and less sugar than processed foods. Patients should be advised to stop adding salt to their food. This may lead to blandness of taste but herbs and spices can be used to help to improve the flavour of food. Occasionally, patients will switch to a salt substitute. This should be discouraged as these are usually very high in potassium and patients with heart failure are likely also to be taking medication, such as ACE-inhibitors and spironolactone, that increases the risk of hyperkalaemia (Good et al. 1995).

Having said all of that, not everyone agrees that patients have to cut down on salt intake if they are not ingesting an excessive amount and the evidence base is weak. There is better evidence suggesting a link between salt and high blood pressure, which should also be avoided in heart failure. The NICE guidelines for chronic heart failure do not give any specific recommendations on salt reduction but the SIGN, ESC and ACC/AHA heart failure guidelines note it as a level C recommendation for patients with advanced heart failure.

Conversely, it is possible for patients to have too little sodium in the blood. Data from the CASTEL study showed that when serum sodium levels are low in the body, the relative risk of death was almost twice that of patients with normal sodium levels (Mazza et al. 2005). Adding sodium as a treatment is not, however, a proven treatment response to low serum sodium.

ALCOHOL

Patients with heart failure and a history of alcoholism need to stop drinking alcohol completely. If they continue to drink, prognosis is poor (Spies et al. 2001). If they stop drinking completely then there can be improvement in cardiac performance (Mølgaard et al. 1990; Jacob et al. 1991). This is because patients with alcoholic cardiomyopathy have more preserved and reversible cardiac function than patients with other dilated cardiomyopathies (Teragaki et al. 1993).

Specialised health teams exist in most areas to help alcoholics stop drinking. There are also well-established self-help groups such as Alcoholics Anonymous – see Box 8.7. As always with lifestyle changes, motivation is the key to success. Non-concordance with abstinence dramatically increases the risk of hospital re-admission among patients with alcoholic cardiomyopathy (Evangelista et al. 2000). Knowing for certain if an alcoholic has stopped drinking is not always straightforward as their self-reporting may be unreliable.

Box 8.7 Alcoholic Support Group Web Link

http://www.alcoholics-anonymous.org.uk/

In heart failure patients who are not alcoholic there are mixed views about whether alcohol should be avoided. It has been argued that all patients with heart failure should abstain from alcohol consumption (Ahmed & Allman 2003). However, several recent, large observational studies found low or moderate alcohol intake did not increase – and sometimes decreased – the risk of heart failure in patients both with and without a previous history of heart failure, of different ages and with or without a history of myocardial infarction (Cooper et al. 2000; Abramson et al. 2001; Aquilar et al. 2004; Klatsky et al. 2005; Salisbury et al. 2005; Bryson et al. 2006).

However, there are a few practical points to make about alcohol intake in heart failure. A large volume of alcohol in a short time, for example binge beer drinking, may precipitate acute decompensation simply through volume overload and this should be avoided. Caution must be exercised in patients taking blood-thinning agents, including beta-blockers, as alcohol will increase clotting time. As excess alcohol is a pro-arrhythmic agent, patients with a history of paroxysmal arrhythmias should avoid alcohol (Djousse et al. 2004; Mukamal et al. 2005).

Box 8.8 Alcohol and Heart Failure Key Messages

- Alcoholics with heart failure must stopping drinking completely.
- Patients with heart failure who drink small or moderate amounts of alcohol (less than 21 units per week for a man and 14 for a woman) can continue to do so but with caution if they have a history of arrhythmias or they are taking blood thinning agents.

SMOKING

There is no known direct causal link between smoking and heart failure as there is for alcohol. There is no doubt, however, about the link between smoking and arteriosclerosis, and up to two-thirds of patients develop heart failure as a result of myocardial infarction. There are also numerous short- and long-term negative haemodynamic effects of smoking, such as increased heart rate, decreased stroke volume, increased blood pressure, increased systemic vascular resistance, increased pulmonary artery pressure, decreased myocardial oxygen delivery and coronary vasoconstriction (Nicolozakes et al. 1988).

It is advisable that all patients with heart failure stop smoking. One study has shown that in patients with heart failure, stopping smoking has a similar mortality benefit to that of drug treatment with ACE-inhibitors, beta-blockers and spirono-lactone (Suskin et al. 2001). The cardiovascular benefit of stopping smoking occurs rapidly, with a 50 % reduction in cardiovascular disease (CVD) risk within one year and an almost normal CVD risk within three years of quitting (Lightwood & Glantz 1997).

Stopping smoking is notoriously difficult and patients with heart failure who smoke are likely to have ingrained lifestyle habits. That said, most patients who smoke do wish to quit and a medical imperative to stop smoking is often a good trigger to begin the process. There has been a great increase in supportive services for people wishing to quit and all local areas will have Smoking Cessation teams to which the patient can be referred, should they so wish.

Box 8.9 Smoking and Heart Failure Key Message

- All patients with heart failure should stop smoking.

STRESS, ANXIETY AND DEPRESSION

Many patients want to know if their heart failure has been caused by stress. By stress, they mean emotional stress. This is difficult to answer, as emotional stress is difficult to quantify or isolate for research purposes. The idea that certain categories of patients (Type A personalities) are more likely to develop cardiovascular disease was a popular theory from the 1950s that seeped into the general consciousness, as it appeared logical and to fit the presentation of heart disease as it was understood at the time.

It is difficult to see how stress could cause chronic heart failure. Physiologically, emotional stress causes a release of neurohormones, which stimulate the heart. In this sense, emotional stress acts like physical stress, as a form of exercise, and so it may actually be beneficial. Theoretically, a chronic stimulation may be harmful, but in actuality it is doubtful as stress tends to be episodic. Stress might be more usefully noted as a possible manifestation of anxiety or depression, both of which are known to be prevalent amongst patients with heart failure and certainly can be a contributory factor to multifactorial symptoms such as dyspnoea (Ramasamy et al. 2006). It is known that depression is an independent predictor of poor outcomes in patients with heart failure (Rumsfeld et al. 2005). What is less clear is whether interventions can mediate this effect.

Patients and relatives who ask whether stress has caused the heart failure invariably do so because the patient has felt, or has seemed to be, under stress. It is a convenient explanation. Clinicians should be wary of giving credence to these beliefs because it may make the patient think that the only treatment they need is to remove the stress. Also, it can confirm conflict within families if one member is blamed for creating the stressful situation.

9 Exercise Training

Exercise training is now recognised as an important component of heart failure treatment. In this chapter the rationale for the use of exercise is explained and the clinical trial data supporting its use are outlined. There is discussion about the practical difficulties of setting up, funding and running exercise programmes, as well as getting patient agreement to participate.

BACKGROUND

A question that many patients with heart failure ask is *'Should I exercise?'*, or alternatively, *'Is it all right for me to exercise?'* This question actually has two parts: firstly, is it helpful to exercise, and secondly, is it safe to exercise? Expert advice on the matter has done a complete about-turn over the past thirty years – from a clear *'no'* to a positive *'yes'*.

The traditional response from health professionals to patients with heart failure was to *'take it easy'*. This is also the assumption by many patients and their carers about what they should do when they have heart failure. The rationale for this is that as the heart is damaged it is best not to put an additional strain on it. This viewpoint seems to be confirmed by the observation that when the patient does exercise they feel fatigued and often breathless. Historically, clinicians went even further and advised patients with more symptomatic heart failure to have a period of bed rest. This was advised because bed rest was thought to rest the heart while allowing better venous return and improving diuresis.

During an episode of severe acute heart failure, a period of bed rest is still advisable in order to reduce haemodynamic strain. However, patients are not generally in acute heart failure very often or for long and once they have recovered, advising bed rest is now thought to show a misunderstanding of the physiology of the heart and the pathophysiology of heart failure. Inactivity leads to reduced exercise tolerance levels and progressive worsening of exertional symptoms (Mancini et al. 1992; McElvie et al. 1995). Common sense tells us that all muscles need to be exercised to stay toned and heart failure is, of course, failure of the heart muscle.

This is not to say that people with heart failure should be advised to enter marathons or to go on climbing holidays in the mountains. Rather, clinicians should be encouraging patients gradually and progressively to increase their activities as by doing so, their exercise tolerance will increase, activities will become easier and their symptoms will improve. This can be done informally by the patient but will be more effective if they can be referred to an exercise training programme.

Cardiac rehabilitation exercise training programmes have existed for some years for patients requiring cardiac rehabilitation following myocardial infarction or after cardiac surgery. As myocardial infarctions, by definition, involve heart muscle death, these patients have some degree of heart failure, even if they are not symptomatic of heart failure. Exercise training for cardiac rehabilitation has been studied extensively over the years.

The usual cardiac rehabilitation exercise training programmes have some limitations for chronic heart failure patients. Firstly, not all patients with heart failure, as we have seen, have a background of ischaemic heart disease. These patients have often been denied access to rehabilitation programmes. A second issue is that traditionally, some rehabilitation programme managers have felt that patients with known heart failure were too high risk to undergo exercise training. There have often been restrictions on access to programmes based on left ventricular ejection fraction because of this belief (Thompson et al. 1997). This exclusion does not stand up to scrutiny, as patients with the worst ejection fractions often have the most to gain and do not have a higher rate of complications during exercise (Erbs et al. 2003). The final problem for patients with heart failure is that exercise training programmes run through cardiac rehabilitation centres are often short in duration (< 12 weeks) whereas the evidence is that heart failure patients benefit most from longer periods of exercise training (Tenenbaum et al. 2006).

EXERCISE PHYSIOLOGY

When exercising, the metabolic demands of the body's tissues rise: there is a need for more oxygen and other nutrients to be delivered and at the same time for more carbon dioxide, toxins and other by-products to be removed. In healthy people this is met by a commensurate rise in cardiac output – up to six times the resting blood demand is possible. As the body exercises it reaches a point where oxygen uptake is at its maximum (known as VO_2max or MVO_2). At 80–95 % of VO_2max excessive build-up of carbon dioxide begins, leading to limitations in oxygen delivery, anaerobic muscle metabolism and lactate production, and resulting in fatigue. A rise in blood carbon dioxide produces arterial acidosis, detected by chemoreceptors, which stimulate hyperventilation and lead to breathlessness.

In patients with heart failure, resting cardiac output may be normal but the ability of cardiac output to increase on exertion is likely to be limited. Their VO_2max will be lower and the physiological response to maximal exercise will be initiated earlier than for someone with an unimpaired heart. Breathlessness that is provoked or made worse on limited exertion is an important symptom indicating heart failure. Stable, well-treated patients may be able to exercise well as the muscle blood flow is maintained at the expense of vasoconstriction in other vascular beds. Patients with heart failure but who are asymptomatic may appear to have normal exercise function in everyday life but may in fact have up to a 30 % reduction in exercise capacity when tested.

As well as VO_2max it is possible to assess exercise function in other ways. Oxygen uptake is also measured by metabolic equivalents (METs): 1 MET is oxygen uptake at rest; activities of daily living generally are about 5 METs; in athletes, METs can be as high as 20. Sub-maximal testing to a predetermined heart rate is often preferred to maximal testing as it is a better indicator of ability to perform activities of living. Tests such as a six-minute walk have the advantage of providing a simple, measurable and repeatable estimation of exercise tolerance. Even asking what activities patients can do is useful as certain activities, such as climbing stairs, require a sudden large increase in cardiac output.

There are several other mechanisms that affect the exercise response of patients with heart failure. Oxygen delivery and utilisation depends upon lung diffusion capacity, transportation via circulation, peripheral perfusion and diffusion, and mitochondria cell function. Respiratory muscles are often abnormal in patients with heart failure (Meyer et al. 2001). In patients with low cardiac output the pulmonary bed is also underperfused. Early muscle deoxygenation, respiratory muscle fatigue and histological changes have all been described. These mechanisms may contribute to the sensation of dyspnoea.

The principal exercise-limiting factor in patients with heart failure often appears to be in the inability of the peripheral, especially leg, muscles to accept more blood. In patients with heart failure, abnormalities have been found in peripheral blood flow, endothelial function and skeletal muscle. It is thought that these abnormalities are linked to a persistent vasoconstrictor drive, relative paucity of peripheral blood vessels, too little nitrous oxide, early lactate release and deficient skeletal muscle metabolism in patients with heart failure (Sinoway 1988). Interestingly, endothelial dysfunction is also believed to be an important factor in hypertension, arteriosclerosis and diabetes mellitus – important and frequent co-morbidities.

RATIONALE FOR EXERCISE TRAINING

After considering the abnormal changes to exercise responses in heart failure, researchers began to consider whether any of these processes could be slowed, stopped or turned around through exercise training. The changes seen in patients with heart failure are in some ways similar to those seen in general physical deconditioning and these are at least partly reversible with exercise training.

There have been several hypotheses as to the mechanisms by which exercise training could work – see Box 9.1. It is likely that exercise training works by a combination of these factors.

Box 9.1 How Does Exercise Training Work?

- down-regulation of neurohormonal responses
- better heart rate variability
- reductions in blood pressure
- improved peripheral tissue perfusion
- reduction in obesity
- positive psychological effects

We have seen in Chapter 5 how patients with heart failure have chronic over-activation of the neurohormonal systems. In Chapter 10 we will consider how many of the drug therapies in heart failure limit this neurohormonal activity. It is believed that exercise training has several effects on these processes. Exercise improves sympathetic nervous tone and responsiveness. Reduced heart rate variability (chronotropic incompetence) is common in heart failure and improved by exercise. Exercise improves peripheral muscle resistance and perfusion (Pu et al. 2001). In patients with heart failure there is impaired regional blood flow and differential shunting of cardiac output during exercise; this can be improved with exercise training. As many of the patients are in a cycle of inactivity and obesity, often with reduced social contacts and self-esteem as a result, the psychological effects of exercise training could also be significant.

EVIDENCE BASE

A number of studies have looked at the safety and efficacy of exercise training in patients with heart failure. These studies have some design weaknesses that have affected the use of their findings. Exercise training is not an intervention that has attracted a lot of research funding and is not of interest to pharmaceutical sponsors so studies have tended to be small in patient numbers and single in site. Small numbers, even in randomised, controlled trial designs, usually mean statistical significance is difficult to achieve. Studies have tended to use a wide variety of types of exercise and duration of training, making comparison of trials sometimes difficult. As there are many unanswered questions as to the importance of the contributions of different mechanisms to the exercise response, these variations may be significant. The use of systematic review and meta-analysis techniques has partly overcome some of the weaknesses in the research designs.

EVIDENCE OF EFFECTIVENESS

It is possible to research several outcomes for exercise training. Symptoms and functional changes can be assessed both subjectively (does the patient feel they can do more?) and semi-objectively (using the NYHA functional scale). Testing can be done to see if exercise tolerance has increased (measuring MVO_2 or exercise treadmill test duration). Echocardiograms can be repeated to look for changes in ejection fraction or contractility. Quality of Life questionnaires can be used along with depression and anxiety scores or other psychological tests. As all of these means are affected by maturation bias – would the patient have become better or worse with the passage of time and disease progression? – it is important that the studies are controlled.

We have noted that patients with heart failure are sometimes offered exercise training as long as they are not in NYHA classes III and IV. This is based on an assumption that these patients are at higher risk of complications or will not be able to manage the programmes. In fact, with supervision and an individualised programme, this is not the case. Logically, patients with the most severe heart failure have the most to gain from improvements. This is borne out by the evidence. In a United States-based study of 68 patients listed for cardiac transplant, who were severely symptomatic with very poor ejection fractions, there was such an improvement in their condition after an exercise programme that 31 of them were removed from the transplant list (Ades 2001).

The benefits of exercise training include symptom improvement and better exercise tolerance (Lloyd-Williams et al. 2002; Beniaminovitz et al. 2002). In one study the average NYHA class fell from 2.4 to 1.3 after 4–6 months of exercise training (Sullivan et al. 1989). That means the average patient in that study went from being symptomatic to asymptomatic.

Objective measures are harder to prove with smaller numbers. In the ELVD-CHF trial, clinical improvements in heart failure with exercise training were also accompanied by improvements in the ejection fraction (Giannuzzi 2003). Improvements in blood count have also been reported in patients with heart failure on exercise programmes (Appleton 2004).

The most important piece of evidence on the benefit of exercise training in heart failure is the meta-analysis in the ExTraMATCH study (Piepoli et al. 2004). The analysis was of nine quality-assessed randomised controlled trials with a total of 801 patients. By pooling the data this study reported, for the first time, a statistically significant benefit to the prognosis for heart failure patients who exercised. In ExTraMATCH, only 17 patients with heart failure had to undergo exercise training in order to save one extra life over two years, compared with the group that underwent standard treatment without exercise training. This was in addition to the benefits to symptoms, exercise tolerance, quality of life and hospitalisation, and possibly also to left ventricular ejection fraction.

Box 9.2 Benefits of Exercise Training in Heart Failure

- symptom improvement – breathlessness, exertional fatigue
- improved quality of life – better mobility and social interaction
- improved left ventricular ejection fraction
- reduced mortality

SAFETY

As we have seen, the traditional advice given to patients with heart failure was not to exercise. As the symptoms of heart failure usually occur on exertion, this was partly to avoid symptoms. Patients or carers often worry that provoking symptoms might lead to new, permanent damage. This is not entirely without justification as there are some reports of left ventricular ejection fraction and wall motion getting worse after exercise in patients with recent acute myocardial infarction. Clinicians were also concerned that because heart failure patients are more vulnerable to arrhythmias and haemodynamic changes, this may make them high risk if they exercised (Kellerman et al. 1988).

In studies that have put patients with heart failure through exercise training, neither arrhythmias nor haemodynamic changes have been shown to occur with any greater frequency than for other patients (Coats et al. 1992; Lloyd-Williams et al. 2002; Appleton 2004). Some studies have even shown a reduced risk of these events (Coats et al. 1992; Belardinelli et al. 1999; Ali et al, 1999).

Even if patients with heart failure are considered higher risk than people without heart failure, it needs to be considered that the alternative to exercising – not exercising – places them at still higher risk of complications and deterioration (North et al. 1990). None the less, it is sensible to minimise risk by ensuring that exercise training programmes are supervised by suitably qualified staff, with emergency procedures in place and access to medical emergency equipment.

CONTRA-INDICATIONS

Some patients should not undergo exercise training. Many of the contra-indications are common sense but others are perhaps less obvious and require knowledge of the patient's history and investigations.

If a patient is physically or mentally unfit to participate in exercise, then they should not do so. As the heart failure population tends to be an elderly one there will be a number of patients with joint or muscle problems or suffering from dementia. This is a safety concern, as exercise training will involve gym equipment and stress testing, both of which require co-ordination and co-operation. That is not to say these patients cannot do some exercise; they should be encouraged to maintain or increase what they are already managing in everyday life. Upper body exercises are possible for even the wheelchair-bound and patients with dementia are often strong walkers.

Patients who have a history of exercise-induced angina or arrhythmias are generally excluded from exercise training programmes. An exception to this rule is patients with refractory angina as there is some evidence that by exercising, collateral coronary blood vessels are built up (Erbs et al. 2006). Patients who experience new exercise-induced angina or arrhythmias should be referred back to the cardiology team for assessment, further investigations and treatment.

Conditions that affect the ability of the heart to eject blood into circulation – such as severe aortic stenosis or left ventricular outflow tract obstructions – preclude exercise because the haemodynamic changes on exercise mean that patients might have angina, a blackout or collapse. Similarly, patients who have conditions that affect the ability of the myocardium to relax, such as amyloidosis, should not undergo exercise training.

Concerns over abnormal haemodynamic responses to exercise mean that it is generally recommended that patients with symptomatic orthostatic hypotension and uncontrolled hypertension should not undergo exercise training until these conditions are better controlled.

The final contra-indications are perhaps obvious – patients who are acutely unwell with either decompensated heart failure or any other systemic illness (such as an acute infection or anaemia) are unsuitable for exercise training at that time. Once treated and stabilised they could then re-enter the exercise-training programme.

Patients have been safely exercised while on ACE-inhibitors and beta-blockers and there are no indications to stop these medicines in order to exercise (Meyer et al. 1991; Demopoulus et al. 1997).

Age is not a contra-indication, although sometimes patients or their carers may perceive it to be so. In fact, analysis of the evidence base suggests the elderly are as likely to gain benefits as younger patients (Fleg 2002).

Box 9.3 Contra-Indications to Exercise Training

- physical incapacity
- mental incapacity
- exercise-induced angina
- exercise-induced arrhythmias
- aortic stenosis and left ventricular outflow tract obstructions
- myocarditis, amyloidosis or fibrosis
- uncontrolled hypertension (systolic > 200; diastolic > 110)
- symptomatic orthostatic hypotension
- acute illness
- decompensated heart failure

TYPES OF EXERCISE TRAINING

There are a number of different ways in which exercise training can be implemented. Various types of exercise using different muscle groups for different periods of exertion, with different haemodynamic targets and varying programme durations have been used. Endurance training is less likely to be tolerated than interval training for patients with chronic fatigue. The research gives no clear answers yet as to what exercise training is best for patients with heart failure. It does seem that the longer the exercise training programme the more significant and sustained the benefits for heart failure patients (Piepoli et al. 1998a, 2004; Demopoulus et al. 1997).

There may be a plateau effect after a quarter to half a year in terms of further improvements but continuing the training should at least maintain the improvements.

Low intensity training is often recommended for patients with heart failure on the assumption that there are still good benefits, while any potential adverse effects from wall stress and negative remodelling are eliminated.

Cycling has been suggested to be more helpful for patients with heart failure than an exercise treadmill. This is because it can be maintained at suboptimal levels for longer and be used by frailer patients. On the other hand, for most patients cycling is less related to daily living than walking.

The European Society of Cardiology recommends interval or endurance training at 40–80 % of peak heart rate, starting with a daily session of 5–10 minutes for four weeks, followed by sessions three to five times a week lasting 20–30 minutes. The guidelines emphasise the importance of continuing with exercise and that inactivity of more than three weeks will lead to the loss of any gains.

SERVICE DELIVERY

The NICE guidelines recommendation R12 advises exercise training – see Box 9.4. Sadly this recommendation is not as strong as it could be and perhaps reflects the fact that the guideline was published before the ExTraMATCH study published its results on the prognostic benefits of exercise training for heart failure patients. Providing exercise training to patients with heart failure also conforms to other government public health agendas, such as reduction in obesity. As a result, there is much interest in exercise programmes and a number of services have been developed.

Box 9.4 NICE Recommendation R12 on Exercise Training in Heart Failure

'Patients with heart failure should be encouraged to adopt regular aerobic and/or resistive exercise. This may be more effective when part of an exercise programme or a programme of rehabilitation.'

It is possible to deliver exercise training in a number of ways: informally or formally; through the NHS, charities or private providers; in secondary care or primary care; and short or long term. Although different models of service all have their advocates it may be that the plurality reflects the different needs of different communities.

Certainly a degree of practicality is needed for people wishing to set up or run exercise training programmes for people with heart failure. A stand-alone heart failure exercise training programme may not be the only or best option. Look at what facilities are already available and make the most of them to minimise start-up costs and use expertise that is already in place and can be transferred. In practice, this usually means expanding cardiac rehabilitation services for ischaemic heart disease patients to include all heart failure patients. This model has been tried and can certainly work (Austin et al. 2005). However it may not be ideal as patients' pathways may not always be similar and they will differ as demographic groups, so some adjustments may be needed.

Home-base programmes are an option. However, success is likely to be tempered by concordance, which in turn is dependent on motivation. One study suggested benefits were only seen if the patients were compliant with the regime for more than 60 % of the time (Hambrecht et al. 1997).

If new facilities or capacity is needed then a business case will need to be made to justify the expenditure. Involving private partners or charities can help to increase participation as well as making a contribution to costs.

Even if no formal exercise training programme is practicable, something can be done. As a minimum, patients should be encouraged to stay active or become active. They should be advised to avoid bed rest and any belief that exercise is harmful should be addressed. Carers should be included in this as they are often the ones advising patients to stop activities and worrying when the patient becomes breathless on exertion. Patients can do much to improve their exercise levels themselves – they can be advised on graded home walking programmes and how to increase their exercise levels in everyday life. For example, a simple way to walk more is to stop parking as close as possible to shop doors but instead to park further away. The British Heart Foundation has leaflets available that reinforce advice on exercising.

BUSINESS CASE

Having made the case that exercise training should be seen as an integral part of heart failure provision, the fact remains that this is an ideal rather than a reality in many areas at present. New monies, or re-allocation of budgets, may be needed to fund an exercise programme and for this a business case will need to be made to the service commissioners.

A business case needs to contain several elements: why the change is needed, how much it will cost to set up, how much it will cost to run, what the savings will be and the costs of not encouraging change. The business case for exercise training in heart failure is compelling.

The evidence base for the efficacy of exercise training in ExTraMATCH is clear. The mortality impact, of only seventeen patients needed for treatment over two years in order to save one life, compares favourably with other forms of treatment (Piepoli et al. 2004). ExTraMATCH also reported a significant reduction in patients' symptoms. It is reasonable to assume this will reduce hospital admissions – this too was found in the ExTraMATCH analysis – and GP attendance. As each heart failure hospital admission costs several thousand pounds, it is easy to see how any reduction quickly saves money. It is also logical to suppose that the benefits may have a positive impact on some patients' ability to return to work, with benefits to the wider economy.

The cost of delivering exercise training depends on whether a service has to be set up from scratch. Even if it does, many facilities that can be used on a sessional basis will already be in place, such as gyms. The biggest costs will mainly be for staff. Even a large programme is unlikely to have hundreds of patients at once and most staff will only need to dedicate a part of their time to the programme. The most cost-effective model is to expand existing cardiac rehabilitation services to take heart failure patients for exercise training. If this is put into effect, the additional costs will probably be only a few thousand pounds per year.

In comparison with all other heart failure interventions, such as medications, devices and surgery, the cost of exercise training is low. It is also tolerated well by patients and has a high success rate and high patient satisfaction levels.

BARRIERS TO CHANGE

While more widespread use of exercise training for heart failure patients is advocated, it is sensible to acknowledge that such services are provided only patchily across the United Kingdom and that there have been barriers to setting up these services.

Lessons can be learned from the slow introduction of cardiac rehabilitation for patients after myocardial infarction. These services were set up largely due to the efforts of committed change agents (Thompson et al. 1997). As a result, the services have varied across the country with regard to where they were based and what they offered. Also, funding for cardiac rehabilitation services has often been *ad hoc* and non-recurrent. Some areas have battled for ongoing funding and have had to incorporate charities and volunteers as well as carrying out their own fundraising. This is in some ways regrettable as the business case for the service is strong. However, the value of cardiac rehabilitation is now well-established.

This difficult history also explains why some cardiac rehabilitation services are concerned about taking on heart failure patients for exercise training. They are worried that their workload will increase without any further resources or funding being put in place to support them. In fact, as we have seen, many of their existing patients have heart failure. The extra numbers referred for exercise training are unlikely to be large, as not all heart failure patients will wish to participate or be capable of doing so.

Arguably, the most important barrier to the use of exercise training in heart failure is the patients themselves or their carers. They may not be able to understand the benefits or they may be expecting instant results; perhaps they believe they are too old or too ill to benefit; or perhaps they don't think it is important. All of these objections are usually surmountable. However, sometimes patients use them as excuses when they just do not want to exercise. If, after explaining the benefits of treatment, a patient does not want to try it then that is their right. Of course, the door should be kept open, in case they change their mind.

10 Medicines

In this chapter the various medications used to treat heart failure and the evidence base supporting their use are presented by drug class. Practical considerations, including side-effects and difficulties in achieving optimal doses, are discussed. Higher risk and problematic patient subgroups are considered. Medications that can worsen heart failure are also noted.

OVERVIEW

Medicines are a mainstay of heart failure management. They can have a positive impact on symptoms, quality of life and prognosis. There have been many developments in the pharmacological treatment of heart failure over the past 30 years and there is now an extensive evidence base supporting most of the various medicines used. Due to the good evidence base, strong recommendations are made in professional heart failure guidelines on which medicines to use in which circumstances. In practice, there are often challenges in getting patients on to these medicines and maintaining them safely.

Box 10.1 Useful Medicines in Heart Failure

Drug class	Examples	Purpose in heart failure
Diuretics	*Furosemide* *Bumetanide* *Amiloride* *Bendroflumethiazide* *Metolazone*	• Remove excess fluid • Reduce cardiac pressures
ACE-inhibitors	*Ramipril* *Perindopril* *Enalapril* *Captopril* *Lisinopril*	• Reduce vasoconstrictive action of angiotensin II • Reduce salt and water retention caused by aldosterone and angiotensin II

Box 10.1 (Continued)

Drug class	Examples	Purpose in heart failure
Beta-blockers	*Bisoprolol* *Carvedilol*	• Improve haemodynamics • Improve cardiac remodelling • Reduce arrhythmias
Aldosterone antagonists	*Spironolactone* *Eplerenone*	• Reduce salt and water retention due to aldosterone
Angiotensin II receptor blockers	*Candesartan* *Losartan* *Valsartan* *Irbesartan*	• Reduce vasoconstrictive action of angiotensin II • Reduce salt and water retention caused by aldosterone and angiotensin II
Nitrates	*Isosorbide Mononitrate* *Isosorbide Dinitrate* *Buccal Suscard* *GTN Spray*	• Reduce pressures by vasodilatation
Inotropes	*Digoxin* *Dopamine* *Dobutamine*	• Increase force of heart contraction

GUIDELINES

Studies have shown repeatedly that patients with heart failure have often not been prescribed the most effective drugs or the most suitable dose (Hobbs 2000; Bungard et al. 2001; Galatius et al. 2004). Under-prescribing has been common and various explanations have been advanced for this and are discussed later in the chapter. Considerable variation in the management of heart failure patients with medication has been a potential source of health inequality.

In order to facilitate more standardised treatment, professional guidelines have been written, as has been the case for many conditions. The European Society of Cardiology (ESC) and the American Heart Association/American College of Cardiology (AHA/ACC) have both developed heart failure guidelines (Swedberg et al. 2005; Hunt et al. 2001). Scotland has developed the SIGN guidelines and these have recently been updated (SIGN 2007). In England the NICE guidelines are in place for the treatment of chronic heart failure (NICE 2003). These analyse the evidence to provide evidence-based recommendations for medication management. The various guidelines do not differ a great deal. This is hardly surprising as many of the experts are in close touch and there is a drive to standardise these types of documents. Medications take up the largest sections of all these guidelines. The documents provide a standard against which practice can be audited. They remain guidelines and clinical judgement must of course be used, and patients' individual conditions, circumstances and wishes considered.

Box 10.2 ESC Guidelines Medication Recommendations in Chronic Heart Failure

	Diuretic(s)	ACE-inhibitor	Angiotensin II receptor blocker	Aldosterone antagonist	Beta-blocker	Digoxin
Asymptomatic (NYHA I)	No	Yes	If ACE-I intolerant	After myocardial infarction	After myocardial infarction	If in atrial fibrillation
Symptomatic (NYHA II)	Yes, if fluid retention	Yes	Yes	After myocardial infarction	Yes	If in atrial fibrillation
Worsening symptoms (NYHA III/IV)	Yes	Yes	Yes	Yes	Yes	Yes
End stage (NYHA IV)	Yes	Yes	Yes	Yes	Yes	Yes

TREATMENT PRINCIPLES

Before considering individually the medicines used in heart failure, it is worth considering treatment principles. The first goal is always to do no harm – the patient should not have worse outcomes on the medicine. As heart failure patients are often finely balanced and the medications powerful, with many potential side-effects, this is a serious concern. The second principle is that the medications should be effective for that patient. This does not equate with the drugs being effective in their clinical trials. Effectiveness can vary in a number of ways – see Box 10.3.

Box 10.3 Intended Outcomes
- improve quality of life
- reduce symptoms

Box 10.3 (Continued)

- improve exercise tolerance
- prevent or slow disease progression
- reduce complications
- reduce hospitalisations
- improve prognosis

ELDERLY PATIENTS

Older patients can have particular issues with regard to medications and the majority of heart failure patients are elderly, as discussed in Chapter 2. Surveys have shown repeatedly that the elderly are less likely to receive medication for their heart failure and this raises the question as to whether they are suffering age discrimination.

The principle of doing no harm is one explanation for the under-usage of drugs in older heart failure populations, especially as non-specialists can be wary of using such powerful medications. As older people are more likely to have co-morbidities that may impact on drug metabolism, such as renal or liver dysfunction, this is understandable. There is concern that increased co-morbidities tend to result in polypharmacy as those conditions are also treated. Difficulties with medication concordance, either through physical or mental incapacity, are of more concern in an older patient group (Witham et al. 2004). These are legitimate clinical concerns and all clinicians must take them into consideration. However, it would be wrong and discriminatory to assume that because a person is older these issues automatically apply to them. As always, there is no substitute for a full, individualised assessment of the patient.

In the past, clinical trials have discriminated against the elderly in that older age has often been an exclusion criterion for trials. The justification for this is usually that the trial is trying to limit extraneous variables and older people may have more of these. The counter argument is that excluding older patients means that the trial results are not 'real-life' and cannot be extrapolated to older patients. Most modern trial designs now include older people and use a statistical analysis of demographic data to test for extraneous variables.

The practical response to using dugs in older patients is to aim for the same evidence-based treatments but to make sure that the initial assessment is thorough and to be vigilant for drug side-effects. The regular monitoring of blood pressure, the heart rate and renal function is advised. Whilst considering age as a potential risk factor for deterioration, remember that age is a poor predictor of health due to large variations in the level of fitness and general health of different patients of the same age.

Box 10.4 Notes on Heart Failure Drugs in the Elderly

Diuretics	Hyperkalaemia is more common in the elderly, especially where spironolactone or potassium-sparing diuretics are used. Reduced renal function reduces effectiveness of diuretics.
ACE-inhibitors and angiotensin II receptor blockers	Have been trialled specifically in the elderly without problems.
Beta-blockers	Usually well tolerated. Note the increased incidence of heart block in the elderly – a contra-indication to beta-blockers.
Digoxin	Elderly more vulnerable to digoxin toxicity if they also have renal impairment.
Nitrates	Elderly more vulnerable to effects of hypotension, especially orthostatic hypotension.

ASYMPTOMATIC PATIENTS

Another group with special medication issues are the asymptomatic heart failure patients. These should receive medicines that have prognostic benefits, such as ACE-inhibitors and beta-blockers. They will not need diuretics as they have no symptoms and there is no definite consensus that diuretics have any effect on prognosis. In practice, asymptomatic patients can often be reluctant to start medications. A good explanation of the natural history of the disease and the long-term benefits of the medicines is important if concordance is to be achieved.

NURSING ROLE

The traditional nursing role with medications has been that of administration. This is important in heart failure, as monitoring the patient's condition for drug effectiveness and potential complications is vital. This will include looking out for dose-related side-effects such as hypotension and bradycardia. Conversely, hypertension and tachycardia may demonstrate that either the patient is unwell or the medication is ineffective. Symptom control may be adequate or inadequate and doses may need adjustment. Side-effects are not as common as patients sometimes think but as a large number of patients are using these drugs, side-effects are seen regularly.

It is common in heart failure services for nurses to have an extended role in the up-titration of medicines (through recommendation to the GP based upon protocol or through patient group directions) or, increasingly, the independent prescription of medicines. The extended role has been shown in trials to be particularly effective in achieving optimal doses of drugs in comparison with standard regimes. It also allows for better detection of side-effects and increased patient satisfaction (Stewart & Blue 2001).

Concordance is often an issue and nurses have a crucial role in educating patients about their medicines and assisting in devising a plan that is acceptable to the individual patient. Concordance includes an assessment of both the physical and psychological ability of the patient to adhere to the treatment prescription. Non-concordance is often involved in treatment failure and is a cause of hospital admissions in heart failure (Jaarsma & Dracup 2001). One of the important benefits of a nurse-led follow-up is improvement in patient concordance.

DIURETICS

PURPOSE

Diuretics are given to remove excess fluid or to prevent fluid building up. They can also help to reduce breathlessness even if there is no apparent excess fluid.

MECHANISM OF ACTION

The kidneys filter out toxins from the blood and maintain a healthy fluid balance to avoid dehydration on the one hand and excess fluid retention on the other. In heart failure, cardiac output can fall and if the blood supply to the renal glomerulus is reduced then filtration slows, tubular reabsorption continues (under the influence of the renin-angiotensin-aldosterone hormones) and excess salt and water build up.

Diuretics reduce the reabsorption of sodium and chloride. By doing so, sodium is lost in the urine. Water is attracted to sodium due to the process of osmosis: whenever sodium is retained, so is water. Diuretics thereby cause the loss of sodium and water in the urine – causing patients to urinate more – hence their colloquial name of 'water tablets'.

TYPES OF DIURETICS

Loop diuretics, such as frusemide and bumetanide, inhibit reabsorption of water and salt in the loop of Henle and also increase potassium secretion in the distal tubule. Potassium secretion is more marked with frusemide usage than with bumetanide. Another practical difference is that bumetanide is absorbed almost completely after oral administration, whereas only 60–70 % of frusemide is absorbed, making bumetanide more effective in patients with poor metabolism, such as during end-stage heart failure. The onset of action by loop diuretics is around 30 minutes after oral administration and just minutes if given intravenously. The duration of action is typically 3–6 hours when given orally. Loop diuretics are the most potent diuretics and are recommended for use in patients with moderate or severe symptomatic heart failure. The adverse effects of loop diuretics are hypokalaemia, hyponatraemia, dehydration, hypotension, nausea, gastric disturbances, hypercalcaemia and gout. Very high doses of frusemide given intravenously over too short a time can lead to temporary tinnitus or even deafness.

Thiazide diuretics, such as bendroflumethiazide, are generally weaker diuretics than loop diuretics. They are well absorbed orally and have a slower onset, longer duration and are less potent than loop diuretics. They are used in patients with mild symptomatic heart failure. Thiazides act on the distal tubule and increase the excretion of sodium, chloride, water and potassium. Adverse effects are similar to that of loop diuretics – hypokalaemia, hyponatraemia and dehydration. The duration of action is around 12 hours, so they need to be given only in the morning. The thiazide diuretic metolazone is particularly effective in producing a large diuresis when used in combination with a loop diuretic.

The third category of diuretics is potassium sparing, such as amiloride and triamterene. These increase the excretion of sodium, chloride and water in the distal tubule but excretion of potassium is inhibited. Their diuretic effect is weaker than that of loop diuretics and they are not the preferred choice in heart failure.

Box 10.5 Types and Doses of Diuretics

Class	Other names	Daily doses (min/max)
Loop		
Frusemide	*Lasix (Celltech)*	20–500 mg
Bumetanide	*Burinex (Leo)*	0.5–10 mg
Torasemide	*Torem (Roche)*	5–200 mg
Thiazide		
Bendroflumethiazide	*(Non-proprietary)*	2.5–10 mg
Metolazone	*Metenix 5 (Borg)*	2.5–10 mg
Indapamide	*Natrilix (Servier)*	2.5 mg
Potassium-sparing		
Spironolactone	*Aldactone (Searle)*	12.5–200 mg
Amiloride	*(Non-proprietary)*	2.5–40 mg
Triamterene	*Dytac (Goldshield)*	25–200 mg

POSITIVE EFFECTS

The positive benefits of diuretics are twofold. Diuretics are of use if the patient shows signs of fluid retention and volume overload. In this case, if the patient is acutely unwell the dose of diuretic may need rapid up-titrating to achieve the desired effect and this may be done even more quickly using the intravenous route.

The second benefit is less well understood by patients but is also important. By removing excess water and by causing vasodilatation, the pressure on the heart – the *preload* – is reduced and the heart is not put under as much strain. This can lead to a reduction in breathlessness. For this reason diuretics can be useful even if there is no apparent fluid retention. At high doses, diuretics can also act as arterial dilators with a reduction of afterload.

Box 10.6 Positive Effects of Diuretics

- remove excess fluid retention
- prevent fluid retention
- reduce preload

NEGATIVE EFFECTS

Diuretics have several potential negative effects. Renal dysfunction occurs both as a primary effect on the kidneys and as a secondary consequence of low blood pressure and dehydration. Patients with existing renal dysfunction should use diuretics with caution. Conversely, patients with advanced renal function often need high doses of diuretics in order to stimulate the kidneys. In patients with renal dysfunction the involvement of the renal specialist team is important.

If the diuretic is working, the patient will pass more water and so runs the risk of passing too much and becoming dehydrated. Patients who are dehydrated run the risk of a metabolic disturbance, the exacerbation of conditions such as gout, and acute admissions with effects such as confusion. In practice, the patient is likely to become thirsty and to drink more if they are dehydrating. Patients who are more vulnerable to dehydration tend to be the elderly or otherwise at-risk people.

Hypotension can be induced if diuresis is strong and circulating volume drops. This may be a problem in that it can exacerbate postural hypotension and this is a problem for patients with heart failure, especially in the elderly. Patients complaining of postural dizziness should have their lying and standing blood pressure measured.

As patients pass more water they will also lose electrolytes; hypokalaemia is a potentially serious problem as, like hyperkalaemia, it can lead to arrhythmias. Certain diuretics are potassium sparing and the use of an ACE-inhibitor makes hypokalaemia less likely. Patients taking diuretics should have regular monitoring of their renal function and electrolytes.

Box 10.7 Possible Negative Effects of Diuretics

- dehydration
- electrolyte imbalances
- hypotension

EVIDENCE BASE

Diuretics have been used in the treatment of heart failure for a long time. Diuretic drugs were introduced before the widespread use of large, randomised, controlled trials to assess drug effectiveness. For this reason they have never been trialled extensively and their effectiveness is supported mainly by empirical evidence from widespread usage (Cody et al. 1994).

A systematic review of the existing small trials (total patient number of 525) has suggested that diuretics may improve prognosis (Faris et al. 2006). For this reason it may be best to continue using diuretics even if the patient shows no signs of fluid retention. However, data from the SOLVD trial suggests that the use of diuretics as a stand-alone therapy is associated with increased neurohormonal activity and should be avoided. Also, a recent study raised concerns that using diuretics in class I and class II patients may actually worsen prognosis (Ahmed et al. 2006).

PRACTICAL CONSIDERATIONS

Before starting a diuretic it is important to assess the patient's fluid status – whether the patient has signs and symptoms of either fluid retention or dehydration. It is also important to know if the patient has renal disease and to have a recent result for U&Es and eGFR.

Current heart failure guidelines agree that it is best to start with a loop diuretic in patients with heart failure. Older guidelines suggest that a thiazide can be used for mild heart failure. The dose depends on the circumstances. Wherever possible it is sensible to start with a low dose (such as frusemide 40 mg OD) and up-titrate as necessary, depending on the effect. If the patient is in acute fluid retention a larger dose, using the intravenous route, may be required. If the patient is retaining fluid despite the loop diuretic having been up-titrated to a high dose, then the addition of a thiazide alongside the loop diuretic should produce profound diuresis. Another option, if not already prescribed, is the addition of spironolactone, which will also increase diuresis.

Many patients want to know if they can stop diuretics once they are asymptomatic or once the excess fluid has been removed. This is difficult to answer because of the lack of trial data. Withdrawing diuretics may make symptoms deteriorate and it is best to down-titrate them gradually rather than stop suddenly. It is sensible, though, to consider reducing the diuretic dose as much as possible to prevent renal dysfunction.

Diuretics are a drug class with frequent concordance issues. These are principally around the social inconvenience of taking the tablets and then having to go to the toilet quickly and frequently. Clearly, if patients are planning to travel or to be out in an unfamiliar environment, the need for close proximity to a toilet can be problematic. This can be addressed in several ways. Firstly, the majority of patients will not be so unstable that the diuretics are crucial. These patients can either delay taking the tablets or even miss that day's tablet. If they are delaying taking them they should be advised not to use them after 4 pm otherwise they are likely to need to get up during the night to pass water. A certain amount of forward planning can also help, such as identifying toilets in the area in advance (for example, at cafés, pubs and many high street shops).

The second issue of concordance tends to occur with patients who have been told the purpose of diuretics is to remove water. This is true, but some patients extrapolate from this that they need only take the diuretics if they are actively retaining fluid. This reasoning is problematic. Firstly, it ignores the possible benefit of preventing the build-up of fluid. Secondly, diuretics also act as a vasodilator and have a positive effect in reducing preload (and to a lesser extent afterload), which has a useful effect on breathlessness.

A problem with some patients who retain fluid, especially in end-stage heart failure, is that they become diuretic-resistant. Before applying this label to a patient, it is worth while making sure of their medicine and diet compliance. However, diuretic resistance does seem to be part of the cardiorenal syndrome whereby worsening renal function leads to higher doses of diuretics being needed or even the application of other techniques such as dialysis to remove excess fluid. In acute decompensated heart failure with fluid retention, an effective alternative to diuretics in a hospital setting can be ultra filtration, as shown in the UNLOAD study (Constanzo et al. 2007). This is rarely seen in clinical practice and is not appropriate if a patient is on a palliative pathway.

ACE-INHIBITORS

PURPOSE

Angiotensin converting enzyme (ACE)-inhibitors are used to reduce breathlessness, improve exercise capacity, decrease hospitalisations and improve prognosis. They are effective in patients with both symptomatic and asymptomatic heart failure.

MODE OF ACTION

Chapter 5 discussed how the renin-angiotensin-aldosterone system (RAAS) plays an important role in blood pressure, blood volume and electrolyte balance. The kidney releases renin in response to low renal perfusion, renin converts angiotensinogen to angiotensin I, and angiotensin converting enzyme (ACE) converts angiotensin I to angiotensin II. Angiotensin II is a powerful vasoconstrictor and it also stimulates aldosterone release, aldosterone being a hormone that increases sodium and water retention. Activation of the RAAS is a normal and useful physiological reaction when renal perfusion drops in order to try to maintain pressure. Yet in patients with heart failure it is chronically over-stimulated and a deleterious cycle of excess pressure and fluid retention causes problems.

In patients with heart failure, low cardiac output will lead to chronic activation of the RAAS. This has a number of negative effects. Angiotensin II is a powerful vasoconstrictor and tightening of the arteries leads to increased afterload – the pressure the heart has to work against – so the left ventricle has to work even harder, leading to hypertrophy. As angiotensin II and aldosterone increase the pressure and volume of the fluid returned to the heart, there is an increase in preload, which can lead to increased intracardiac volumes and chamber dilation. The net effect of these high pressures is that fluid is forced out of the blood vessels and into the tissues of the lungs and the peripheries as pulmonary and peripheral oedema.

ACE-inhibitors block the angiotensin converting enzyme (ACE), which converts angiotensin I to angiotensin II. It does this by competitive binding to the receptor. Angiotensin I is essentially inactive but angiotensin II is a powerful agent. As angiotensin II is a vasoconstrictor, blocking it with an ACE-inhibitor leads to vasodilation. By vasodilatation, ACE-inhibitors lower pressures and ease breathlessness. As angiotensin II leads to aldosterone production with salt and water retention, an ACE-inhibitor will also reduce aldosterone production, thereby reducing the mechanism of salt and water retention and increased preload.

As the RAAS cascade is activated in response to low renal blood flow, it might be thought that blocking the RAAS could lead to a decline in renal blood flow. This is partially true in that too high a dose of ACE-inhibitors could lower blood pressure to a dangerous level. However, in the kidneys ACE-inhibitors cause greater dilation of the efferent arterioles than the afferent arterioles, thereby reducing intraglomerular pressure and protecting the kidneys.

POSITIVE EFFECTS

ACE-inhibitors have been shown to have several important benefits in patients with all classes of heart failure. Patients taking ACE-inhibitors are less likely to have symptoms, less likely to be hospitalised for heart failure and more likely to live longer than similar patients who do not take an ACE-inhibitor. This means all patients with heart failure should take ACE-inhibitors, where tolerated.

We noted in Chapter 2 that many patients with heart failure have had a myocardial infarction and in Chapter 5 discussed how, after myocardial infarction, compensatory changes occur, which can result in the remodelling of the left ventricular shape and lead on to heart failure. ACE-inhibitors change this process and therefore should be prescribed to all patients who have had a myocardial infarction, without contra-indications, regardless of whether there is any evidence of heart failure, in order to try to prevent the development of heart failure (The HOPE Study Investigators 2000).

The effects of ACE-inhibitors on symptoms such as breathlessness can sometimes be seen relatively quickly. Other benefits, such as reduced rehospitalisations and better prognosis, are only seen over months or even years.

NEGATIVE EFFECTS

There are several possible problems with ACE-inhibitors. Some are observed fairly frequently, such as a cough and hypotension, while others are unusual, such as rashes and taste disturbance. There are also issues with regard to renal function and electrolyte balance.

The side-effect most widely experienced with ACE-inhibitors is the dry cough. The cough is believed to be a result of ACE-inhibitors being involved in the breakdown of bradykinin. This occurs in the lungs and bradykinin acts as an irritant. This side-effect occurs in around 10–15 % of patients who start ACE-inhibitors. It is a very common reason why patients stop taking ACE-inhibitors. The cough is often temporary so the patient should be encouraged to persist for a few weeks to see if it disappears. If not, angiotensin II receptor blockers offer an acceptable alternative that will not produce a cough as a side-effect.

As they act as vasodilators, ACE-inhibitors lower patients' blood pressure. When ACE-inhibitors were first introduced there was concern that first-dose hypotension may be a significant problem but experience has shown it rarely happens if a sensible-sized first dose is given. ACE-inhibitors may lower the blood pressure for longer periods of time and it is possible for them to lower the blood pressure too much. Should this occur, the patient might experience symptoms such as dizziness, nausea or postural hypotension.

Occasionally patients starting ACE-inhibitors may report a loss of taste, or an abnormal metallic taste, or aphthous mouth ulcers. There are also other rarely occurring side-effects such as self-limiting maculopapular or prucitic rashes early in treatment. Very rarely, patients may have angioedema of the face, lips and larynx.

EVIDENCE BASE

ACE-inhibitors came into practice in the 1980s and their use in heart failure was trialled widely into the 1990s. Box 10.8 outlines the main trials of ACE-inhibitors in heart failure patients.

Box 10.8 ACE-Inhibitor Heart Failure Trials

SOLVD (The SOLVD Investigators 1991)	SOLVD used enalapril and found a reduced rehospitalisation rate as well as mortality and functional improvements.
SAVE (Pfeffer et al. 1992)	SAVE looked at post myocardial infarction patients with asymptomatic heart failure and found captopril improved mortality and morbidity.
CONSENSUS (Kjekshus et al. 1992)	The CONSENSUS study used enalapril and, as well as improved mortality, found treated patients improved functionally (NYHA class), with better exercise tolerance, smaller heart size and less medication use.

Box 10.8 (Continued)

AIRES (The AIRE Study Investigators 1993)	AIRES looked at ramipril in a group of post myocardial infarction patients with heart failure similar to that of SAVE, except these patients were symptomatic, and also found improved survival.
ATLAS (Packer et al. 1999)	The ATLAS trial was important because it looked at lisinopril at different doses and concluded that the higher the dose the better the mortality and rehospitalisation rate.

These randomised, controlled trials of ACE-inhibitors and heart failure contain over 15 000 patients in total and cover a wide spectrum of patients. That said, the elderly are a little under-represented, as has been typical in clinical trials. The trials show a consistent pattern of benefit to ACE-inhibitor use in heart failure. Results showed significant benefits in both symptomatic and asymptomatic patients and ACE-inhibitors are therefore recommended as a first-line essential therapy for all patients with a diagnosis of heart failure, if tolerated. ACE-inhibitors improve prognosis in all patients, although the benefit is more marked in severely ill patients. Exercise capacity improves in patients with depressed left ventricular functions. Higher doses reduced the risk of hospitalisation, in the ATLAS study, but have not been shown to affect mortality or symptoms.

There doesn't seem much to choose between the different types of ACE-inhibitors and it is assumed that they have a class effect in terms of effectiveness and side-effects.

PRACTICAL CONSIDERATIONS

ACE-inhibitors are not suitable for all patients. The contra-indications for ACE-inhibitor use are listed in Box 10.9.

Box 10.9 Contra-indications to ACE-Inhibitors

- severe renal dysfunction (creatinine > 300)
- renal artery stenosis
- hyperkalaemia
- hypovolaemia
- hyponatraemia
- pregnancy or breast feeding
- left ventricular outflow tract obstruction and aortic stenosis
- hypotension
- cor pulmonale
- symptomatic peripheral artery disease

If the patient has no contra-indications to ACE-inhibitor use then they should commence with a low dose. Starting doses and target doses are given in Box 10.10. The goal is to achieve the highest dose possible. To achieve this a process of up-titration is necessary because if the patient is given a high dose straight away they are much more likely to have adverse reactions. The NICE guidelines recommend the ACE-inhibitor be doubled in dose, with a minimum gap of two weeks and a blood test for renal function, until the target dose is reached. Not all patients will achieve full dose – usually because the blood pressure has fallen to a level at which any further blood pressure reduction might be problematic. Not being on the target dose is fine, as long as they have had the opportunity to do so and are on the maximum tolerated dose. It is important to remember that a little ACE-inhibitor is better than none and not to make patients feel they have failed if they do not achieve the target dose – they are on the right amount for them. Nurses have an important role in supervising ACE-inhibitor up-titration as studies show that in the past as few as a third of suitable community patients were taking ACE-inhibitors at the target dose (Cowie & Kirby 2003).

Box 10.10 ACE-Inhibitor Starting and Target Doses

Drug	Proprietary names	Initial dose	Maximum dose
Captopril	Capoten (Squibb)	6.25 mg tds	25–50 mg tds
Enalapril	Innovace (MSD)	2.5 mg od	10 mg bd
Lisinopril	Carace (Bristol-Myers Squibb); Zestril (AstraZeneca)	2.5 mg od	5–20 mg od
Ramipril	Titrace (Aventis Pharma)	1.25–2.5 mg od	2.5–5 mg bd
Perindopril	Coversyl (Servier)	2 mg od	4 mg od (8 mg if hypertensive)
Trandolapril	Gopten (Abbott); Odrik (Hoechst Marion Roussel)	1 mg od	4 mg od

od = once daily
bd = twice daily
tds = three times a day

When a patient begins taking an ACE-inhibitor there is the possibility of first-dose hypotension. For many years these concerns led to patients being admitted to hospital for 'Captopril trials'. Captopril tended to be the ACE-inhibitor used for these trials as it has the shortest half-life. Practice moves on and, with experience, first-dose hypotension became less of an issue in everyday practice than first thought. Most centres no longer hospitalise patients to carry out trials. None the less, it is necessary to warn the patient that hypotension is a possibility and that it is best to take their first dose in the evening on retiring to bed. If patients feel dizzy they should be instructed to lie down and, if this persists, to seek medical advice.

We have seen how ACE-inhibitors lower blood pressure because of their vasodilator effect. Patients taking ACE-inhibitors may be hypotensive but if the patient is asymptomatic then hypotension should not necessitate stopping or reducing the ACE-inhibitor. If the patient is symptomatic, or if their blood pressure is worryingly low (less than 80 mmHg systolic), then the NICE guidelines recommend reducing or stopping other anti-hypertensives, such as nitrates, before the ACE-inhibitor. Hypotension is the second most common reason that ACE-inhibitors are not used, or are reduced or stopped. Non-specialists are especially liable to change or stop using the ACE-inhibitor if they observe low blood pressure. Remember that these patients may be chronically hypotensive due to heart failure or other medications.

If the patient develops a cough after starting an ACE-inhibitor then it is worth asking them to continue as the cough usually goes within a few weeks. The cough will be dry and unresponsive to antitussives. Like any cough, the more they cough the greater the local trauma, and so the situation worsens. If the situation continues or is intolerable for the patient, the ACE-inhibitor will have to be stopped and the patient switched to an angiotensin II receptor blocker. There is no point changing from one ACE-inhibitor to another as the cough is a drug class side-effect.

It is worth remembering that many patients have a cough for many different reasons – sometimes due to paroxysmal nocturnal dyspnoea, but mainly from coincidental throat infections or even for psychogenetic reasons. Find out when the cough began – if it preceded the ACE-inhibitor then logically this is not the cause. It is sometimes worth while, if you are unsure of the sequence of events, to try reintroducing the ACE-inhibitor at a later stage to see if the cough occurs again and if it does, then you can be sure the patient cannot tolerate it. As ACE-inhibitors have important benefits, it is vital that patients can reap the advantages, if at all possible.

Once a patient starts on an ACE-inhibitor their renal function will need to be checked within two weeks. Some deterioration is usual and, if slight, just needs rechecking a few weeks later. If the disturbance is significant (a rise in creatinine of more than 50 % from baseline or an absolute rise to above 300) or the patient is symptomatic then consider reducing their diuretics before the ACE-inhibitor. If their renal function does not recover, specialist renal opinion will be needed. As ACE-inhibitors can cause haematological side-effects it is also worth while checking the blood count. Haematological disturbances will usually be reversible on discontinuation of treatment.

As we have noted, chronic renal dysfunction is not a contra-indication to starting an ACE-inhibitor, as long as the patient does not have severe dysfunction or significant renal artery stenosis. Chronic renal dysfunction is common, especially in the elderly and in patients with co-morbidities such as diabetes. Heart failure as it progresses means the blood supply to the kidneys is reduced and renal dysfunction can occur. It is therefore quite common for patients with heart failure also to have renal dysfunction. As the heart and renal failure worsens it may be necessary to reduce the dose of the ACE-inhibitor.

ANGIOTENSIN II RECEPTOR BLOCKERS (A2RB)

PURPOSE

Angiotensin II receptor blockers work in the RAAS cascade, like ACE-inhibitors, with similar beneficial effects such as reducing symptoms, reducing hospitalisations and improving prognosis.

MODE OF ACTION

Angiotensin II receptor blockers reduce afterload and preload by vasodilation and inhibit aldosterone release, preventing sodium and water retention. There are two classes of angiotensin II receptors: AT1 and AT2. It appears that AT1 receptors are blocked mainly by the current angiotensin II receptor blocker drugs and AT1 receptors are found mainly in the heart, blood vessels, renal cortex, lung and brain. The reasons why angiotensin II receptor blockers do not cause a cough can be seen when looking at the RAAS cascade – see Box 5.5 – in that they do not affect bradykinin breakdown.

POSITIVE AND NEGATIVE EFFECTS

The positive benefits of A2RBs are believed to be equivalent to those of ACE-inhibitors.

EVIDENCE BASE

Angiotensin II receptor blockers have not been trialled as extensively as ACE-inhibitors as they are newer pharmaceutical compounds – see Box 10.11. The only angiotensin II receptor blocker to have received a licence for heart failure in the United Kingdom is candesartan, on the strength of the CHARM trial. Although there may be a class effect for all angiotensin II receptor blockers, this is unproven. Nor is it known if there is a dose effect, although it is assumed that higher doses block more receptors and should be used where possible.

Some studies have considered whether angiotensin II receptor blockers should be used in conjunction with ACE-inhibitors. The CHARM trial showed improved outcomes when this was done. This would provide a more extensive blocking of the RAAS than using a single agent. Certainly, adding an angiotensin II receptor blocker to the ACE-inhibitor is worth while in a patient who continues to be highly symptomatic. Practical issue with adding one in this way is that it increases the polypharmacy of these patients, lowers their blood pressure even further and perhaps puts more of a strain on renal function.

Box 10.11 Trials of Angiotensin II Receptor Blockers

ELITE-1 (Pitt et al. 1997)	A small trial of elderly patients compared losartan with captopril and found that losartan produced lower mortality and was better tolerated than captopril.
RESOLVD (McElvie et al. 1999)	Compared enalapril with candesartan and did not support the findings of ELITE-1.
VAL-HeFT (Cohn & Tognoni 2001)	The VAL-HeFT trial used valsartan versus placebo and also found improvements in mortality along with improvements in symptoms of heart failure.
CHARM (Yusuf et al. 2003)	Large trial of candesartan versus placebo found candesartan to be well tolerated with positive effects on prognosis and admissions.
ELITE-2 (Konstam et al. 2005)	Compared captopril with losartan and the hypothesis that losartan was better than enalapril was not proved.

PRACTICAL CONSIDERATIONS

The main use of angiotensin II receptor blockers currently is as an alternative to ACE-inhibitors in patients who have a persistent and intolerable cough. As they work in a similar manner to ACE-inhibitors, it is logical to treat in a similar manner: start with a low dose and then up-titrate, carrying out renal function and blood pressure checks.

Box 10.12 Starting and Target Doses of Angiotensin II Receptor Blockers

Drug	Proprietary names	Total daily doses
Candesartan	*Amias (AstraZeneca, Takeda)*	4 mg–16 mg
Irbesartan	*Aprovel (Bristol-Myers Squibb, Sanofi-Synthelabo)*	150 mg–300 mg
Losartan	*Cozaar (MSD)*	50 mg–100 mg
Valsartan	*Diovan (Novartis)*	80 mg–320 mg

BETA-BLOCKERS

PURPOSE

Beta-blockers are used to increase the efficiency of the heart's pumping action, reduce arrhythmias and improve the shape of the heart over time.

MODE OF ACTION

As we saw in Chapter 5, the body responds to physiological (or psychological) stress by releasing adrenaline to stimulate the sympathetic nervous system. Beta-adrenaline stimulation increases the heart rate, conduction velocity and the force of myocardial contraction, and causes arterial vasodilation. In patients with heart failure, low cardiac output is compensated for by constant stimulation of the beta-adrenaline receptors and over time this reduces the responsiveness of the myocardium to stimulation. In turn this means even more adrenaline is produced, causing a vicious spiral of deterioration.

Beta-blockers bind competitively to beta-adrenaline receptors. Two types of these receptors are found in the body: the majority of beta-1 receptors are located in the heart, whereas beta-2 receptors are found mainly in the airways, blood vessels and other organs. Some beta-blockers work mainly on beta-1 receptors and are considered more *cardioselective*.

The most obvious effects of blocking beta-receptors are to slow down the heart and to reduce blood pressure. This is helpful in several ways. By slowing the heart (negative chronoptropy) the diastolic filling time is increased, allowing more blood to enter the left ventricle, and improving stroke volume and contractility (positive inotrophy) by the Frank-Starling mechanism. Over time this can lead to positive structural adaptations within the left ventricle. Beta-blockers also act as anti-arrhythmics and this effect is useful in heart failure because as heart failure develops the heart is more arrythmogenic.

POSITIVE EFFECTS

Beta-blockers are an unusual medication in heart failure in that they generally do not make the patient feel any better – at least, not in the short-term. Indeed, in the short-term they often make patients feel worse. They do, however, have clear benefits in the clinical trials regarding mortality and rehospitalisation. Meta analysis shows 3.8 lives saved and four fewer hospitalisations per 100 patients treated in beta-blocked heart failure patients compared with those not on beta-blockers in the first year (Brophy et al. 2001). These are important benefits and most patients are willing to try the drug, even if it is unlikely to improve symptoms immediately.

NEGATIVE EFFECTS

It is common for patients to experience a deterioration in symptoms when first starting beta-blockers or when increasing the dose. Patients often report feeling more fatigued and sometimes more breathless for a few days. This is probably due to the haemodynamic adjustments being made as the body adjusts to the drug. Generally these effects are self-limiting and rarely last for more than a few days. None the less, the patient should be warned that this might happen because if they are not warned, they may think they are having an adverse reaction and stop taking the drug. Most people do not notice anything different when starting a beta-blocker, if the dose is low enough.

A more serious adverse event is bronchospasm, as beta-receptors in the airways are blocked, but this is a rare occurrence when introducing a beta-blocker. If a patient has a history of bronchospasm then a beta-blocker is contra-indicated. In practice, the patient group to be wary of are true asthmatics. Chronic obstructive airways disease is not, however, a contra-indication as in these patients the beta-receptors in the airways are down-regulated over time. Some beta-blockers (acebutolol, atenolol, betaxolol, bisoprolol and metoprolol) are cardioselective – they block the beta-1 receptors at doses small enough not to effect the beta-2 receptors – although it is worth noting that no beta-blockers are absolutely cardiospecific.

Beta-blockers can worsen the symptoms of peripheral vascular disease. A diagnosis of peripheral vascular disease, unless severe, does not contra-indicate the use of beta-blockers but they should be used with caution and with the patient's agreement.

As beta-blockers slow the heart rate, a patient with an abnormally slow heart rate should not be started on a beta-blocker, at least until the cause of the bradycardia is investigated and treated. If the patient is treated with a pacemaker then they can safely take a beta-blocker.

EVIDENCE BASE

Beta-blockers have been used in cardiac patients since the 1960s in order to reduce blood pressure, prevent angina, regulate rhythm and reduce anxiety. They were thought to be contra-indicated in patients with heart failure because of perceived reduction of contractility, until the results of trials in the 1990s demonstrated that far from being harmful, they were in fact very beneficial – see Box 10.13.

Box 10.13 Beta-blocker Heart Failure Trials

COPERNICUS (Packer et al. 1996)	Carvedilol in patients with severe heart failure improved symptoms, rehospitalisation and mortality.
CIBIS-II (The CIBIS-II Investigators 1999)	Bisoprolol improved total mortality by 34 % and reduced sudden death by 40 % over placebo in patients with class III and class IV heart failure.
MERIT-HF (The MERIT-HF Investigators 1999)	Metoprolol improved total mortality by 32 % and sudden cardiac death by 50 % over placebo in patients with classes II, III and IV heart failure.
COMET (Poole-Wilson et al. 2003)	Metoprolol and carvedilol were compared and carvedilol was slightly better at reducing mortality and hospital admissions than metoprolol.

Over 10 000 patients took part in these beta-blocker trials (COPERNICUS, CIBIS-II and MERIT-HF), which showed convincingly that beta-blockers are of benefit to patients with heart failure, especially severe heart failure, producing reductions in mortality, symptoms and hospitalisation. Reduction in heart failure hospitalisation was not accompanied by a rise in all-cause admissions.

These benefits are probably produced by a combination of the drug's actions on haemodynamic, remodelling and rhythm control. It is not known whether there is a class effect for beta-blockers but it is thought to be likely that there are some differences between different beta-blockers. Carvedilol, for example, also has some alpha-adrenaline-blocking effects, which may account for its better effectiveness when compared with metoprolol in the COMET trial. In all the trials the beta-blockers had a short-term negative inotropic effect but after three months there were improvements in left ventricular systolic function. After longer treatment, ventricular shape normalisation and regression in myocardial hypertrophy – *reverse modelling* – can be seen in some treated patients. Some trials have shown a significant improvement in exercise tolerance, whereas others report no change or a negative change.

In the United Kingdom the only two beta-blockers licensed for use in heart failure are carvedilol and bisoprolol. The NICE guidelines leave it up to the clinician to decide which to use. Bisoprolol is more beta-1 cardioselective whereas carvedilol has some alpha-blocking effects. The guideline does suggest that if a patient is already taking a different beta-blocker (such as atenolol for angina) then there is probably no overwhelming reason to change their prescription. In other countries other beta-blockers, especially metoprolol, are used in heart failure.

The results of trials that looked at the quality of life of heart failure patients who take beta-blockers are conflicting. The MDC trial (Waagstein et al. 1993) showed an improvement in quality of life whereas the RESOLVD (McKelvie et al. 1999) and US Carvedilol trials (Colucci et al. 1996) showed no change while the Australian-New Zealand Study (The Australia-New Zealand Heart Failure Research Collaborative Group 1995) showed a declining quality of life for patients who were taking beta-blockers. This information fits with clinical experience and indicates that the purpose of treatment should be discussed with patients – if quality of life is a priority rather than longevity, then a high dose of beta-blockers may not be ideal for that patient.

There are some gaps in the information the beta-blocker trials provided. The trials included patients with chronic, symptomatic heart failure of both ischaemic and dilated cardiomyopathy backgrounds. However, it is unclear whether patients with diastolic dysfunction or valvular heart failure will benefit from beta-blockers as these patients were not included. The same applies to patients with class I heart failure. Class IV patients were also under-represented in the trials. The COPERNICUS trial did include class IV patients and found they benefited from beta-blockers but this subgroup did not involve a large number of patients. A United States trial, BEST, with a large Afro-American sample, found beta-blockers to be less effective than in studies with a largely Caucasian sample. This may suggest some racial differences of clinical significance as Afro-Americans also tend to have a higher incidence of hypertension and in hypertension trials they respond less well to standard treatment.

PRACTICAL CONSIDERATIONS

Beta-blockers are now recommended by all of the guidelines for all suitable patients needing treatment for heart failure. However, not everyone is considered suitable and not everyone can tolerate the drugs, or not necessarily at optimal doses; nor does everyone agree to take them.

There are some definite contra-indications to using beta-blockers (such as a history of bronchospasm, severe peripheral vascular disease and previous allergic reactions) and caution is advised for many patients, such as those with chronic obstructive pulmonary disease and hypotension. Whether heart failure patients get beta-blockers has in the past often depended on how bold clinicians are with regard to the caution advised and how ready they are to stop the drugs if potential side-effects occur. Studies have reported ineligibility rates for beta-blockers of 20 % (Witham et al. 2004), 43 % (Mahmudi et al. 2003) and 31 % (Baxter et al. 2002). It is worth clinicians remembering, on the positive side, the proven mortality benefits of beta-blockers.

When starting heart failure patients on beta-blockers, the NICE guidelines recommend specialist supervision, although they do not indicate how close this should be, while the drug manufacturers' guidelines recommend blood pressure is checked for four hours after the first dose. In practical terms most clinicians have taken this to mean hospital supervision, usually in an investigation unit, day case unit or outpatient observation ward. The concerns are for bronchospasm and first dose hypotension but these are extremely rare, especially if patients are assessed well beforehand and a low beta-blocker dose is used. It is likely that admitting patients for beta-blocker trials will eventually decline in the same way that admitting patients for captopril trials has. There is no reason why, with services in place, beta-blockers cannot be initiated in the community for the majority of heart failure patients.

Intolerance of beta-blockers is often the result of the dosage. If a patient receives an initial dose that is too high they may well become symptomatically hypotensive or bradycardic. The rule to remember is 'start low, go slow'. If a patient says they are intolerant of beta-blockers, a little detective work to find out what went wrong, which drug was used and in what dosage, may reveal that they were given too ambitious a dose and that they perhaps might tolerate a more cautious regime.

Beta-blockers are most effective at higher doses for heart failure. Achieving this is difficult on both clinical and practical grounds. Clinically it is difficult because heart rate and blood pressure often drop to a level where any further dose increases may provoke symptoms. When this point is reached the patient is on the maximum *tolerated* dose and this will vary among patients. Practically, achieving higher doses can be problematic, as someone needs to take responsibility for arranging regular follow-ups to check the patient and carry out up-titration.

The up-titration process can be a lengthy one. The NICE guidelines recommend doubling the dose at not less than two-weekly intervals. Increasing the number of steps and the gaps between up-titration is more likely to increase tolerance. For example, bisoprolol is available in tablets of 1.25 mg, 2.5 mg, 3.75 mg, 5 mg, 7.5 mg and 10 mg and these are the steps that many clinicians will use, with gaps of four weeks in between up-titration. If the process is being supervised in a clinic then the practicalities of clinic slots and processes may influence the regime. Up-titration can be supervised in the community although research shows this is still best overseen by a specialist, as leaving the process to general practitioners tends to lead to under-dosing.

Box 10.14 Beta-blocker Starting and Target Doses

Non-proprietary name	Proprietary name	Starting dose	Target dose
Bisoprolol	*Cardicor (Merck); Emcor (Merck); Monocor (Lederle)*	1.25 mg OD	10 mg OD
Carvedilol	*Eucardic (Roche)*	3.125 mg OD	50 mg OD (twice daily if the patient weighs more than 85 kg)

Beta-blockers are under-prescribed for a variety of reasons. Some clinicians recall that beta-blockers were contra-indicated in heart failure in the past and they still have reservations about using them. Others have concerns about potential cautions and side-effects. It is certainly true that it takes careful monitoring and persistence to achieve the optimal doses, that the optimal dose is often not the maximal, and that ineligibility and side-effects are more common in clinical practice than in trials.

A practical concordance issue with bisoprolol is that the dosages appear small – for example, 1.25 mg OD. This is slightly misleading as it is the equivalent of higher doses of atenolol or metoprolol. Occasionally patients undergoing up-titration believe that they can speed up the process and so they increase the doses themselves. Anecdotally, this seems to happen more frequently with men than women. The patient may or may not have any problems as a result but they should be encouraged to stick to the up-titration regime.

ALDOSTERONE ANTAGONISTS

PURPOSE

The purpose of aldosterone antagonists is to reduce symptoms such as breathlessness and improve prognosis in patients with severe heart failure.

MODE OF ACTION

As we saw in Chapter 5, aldosterone is a hormone released as part of the renin-angiotensin-aldosterone system. Aldosterone acts within the distal tubule of the kidney to retain sodium and water. Blocking aldosterone means that less sodium and water is retained and more is excreted. Conversely, more potassium is retained. Aldosterone antagonists act as potassium-sparing diuretics.

POSITIVE EFFECTS

Aldosterone antagonists reduce the preload pressures on the heart. This can lead to a symptomatic improvement in patients who are breathless. Data from the RALES trial showed that patients with NYHA class III and class IV heart failure who took spironolactone had a better prognosis than those who did not (The RALES Investigators 1996). This is thought to be due to a similar mechanism by which ACE-inhibitors improve prognosis in patients with heart failure.

NEGATIVE EFFECTS

There are two side-effects to aldosterone antagonism that are seen reasonably frequently in clinical practice and often lead to the drug being stopped.

As the drug acts as a potassium-sparing diuretic it is possible that too much potassium is retained and the patient may become hyperkalaemic. Any substantial changes outside of the relatively tight normal serum potassium range can lead to arrhythmias. Hyperkalaemia is also a possible side-effect of ACE-inhibitors, which the patient is likely to be taking in addition to the aldosterone antagonist. Whilst hyperkalaemia is not common it is more likely to occur in the elderly and patients with coexisting renal disease, both of which are often characteristic of patients with heart failure.

Swollen, painful breast tissue (gynaecomastia) is a hormonal side-effect. In the RALES trial up to 10 % of the men taking spironolactone developed gynaecomastia up to three months after starting treatment. This is often intolerable for male patients for both comfort and body image reasons and the spironolactone may have to be stopped. The new aldosterone antagonist, eplerenone, does not seem to produce gynaecomastia but as yet is only licensed in the United Kingdom for post myocardial infarction heart failure.

EVIDENCE BASE

The evidence base supporting aldosterone antagonist drugs in heart failure is much less extensive than that for other medications. There has been only one randomised controlled trial of spironolactone in heart failure, the RALES trial, and one trial of eplerenone, the EPHESUS trial (Pitt et al. 2005).

The RALES trial used spironolactone in patients with severe heart failure and found an improvement in mortality, symptoms and re-admissions. The trial contained less than 2000 patients and did not involve patients with mild or asymptomatic heart failure. Spironolactone can only be recommended in patients with NYHA class III or IV heart failure with a left ventricular ejection fraction of less than 35 %.

Hyperkalaemia occurred rarely in the RALES trial. That aspect of the RALES results has been questioned following the results from a study in Toronto, Ontario, which showed that the risks of hyperkalaemia were much higher in a typical heart failure population taking spironolactone than those in the RALES trial – with hospital admissions through hyperkalaemia offsetting any reduced heart failure admissions due to the beneficial effects of spironolactone (Juurlink et al. 2004). It is worth noting, though, that hypokalaemia is also a serious potential risk and spironolactone would help to protect the patient against this.

A second study of aldostreone antagonists has recently been undertaken. This is the EPHESUS trial using eplerenone. In the trial eplerenone was found to produce beneficial effects similar to spironolactone in terms of symptoms and mortality. This drug has the considerable advantage of not causing gynaecomastia. The EPHESUS trial population was patients with heart failure immediately following a myocardial infarction, the use for which it has been licensed in the United Kingdom. If the drug was to be used for chronic patients as a substitute for spironolactone, this would be off-licence at present.

PRACTICAL CONSIDERATIONS

Although a diuretic, spironolactone has an onset time of around two to four hours, so it is less likely to cause patients to dash to the lavatory than a diuretic such as frusemide. It would be sensible not to take the drug too late in the day to avoid excessive nocturnal diuresis. The duration of spironolactone can be fairly long – up to four days – so it can take several days to observe a beneficial effect on symptoms and to clear from the system if the patient is hyperkalaemic.

Before starting a patient on spironolactone it is important to check their baseline renal function with blood tests. Then repeat the blood tests a week to ten days after starting the drug. A rise in potassium level of up to 6 mmol/l is seen as acceptable in most guidelines. Hyperkalaemia would need to be much higher than that to lead to arrhythmias. If a patient has a potassium level above that amount, spironolactone should be stopped at least temporarily until the level returns within the normal range, and then restarted at a lower dose.

If the patient complains of gynaecomastia then their symptoms are unlikely to resolve without ceasing spironolactone. The patient would then miss out on the beneficial effects of the drug. A patient may be willing to tolerate some enlargement but is less likely to be able to continue with the drug if the breasts are also tender. Unfortunately, even after stopping the drug it can take some time for the symptoms to improve.

Box 10.15 Aldosterone Antagonists – Key Messages

- Patients with NYHA class III or IV heart failure with LVEF < 35 % should be prescribed spironolactone.
- Patients post AMI in heart failure should be prescribed eplerenone.
- Patients on aldosterone antagonists need regular potassium monitoring.

DIGOXIN

PURPOSE

Digoxin is given to improve the contractility (positive inotrope) of the heart and to slow down its speed (negative chronotrope). By doing so, cardiac output is improved without raising filling pressures.

MODE OF ACTION

Digoxin is a cardiac glycoside that inhibits sodium transport out of cells, affecting intracellular calcium levels. As calcium affects myocardial contractility digoxin is a positive inotrope, increasing the force of contraction. It is also a negative chronotrope – slowing down the heart – because it increases vagal nerve tone, decreasing the automaticity of the sinoatrial node and conduction velocity of the atrioventricular node, thereby prolonging the refractory period.

POSITIVE EFFECTS

If a patient has an abnormally fast heart rate then slowing it down can make them feel better as they should have fewer palpitations, less breathlessness and possibly less chest pain. Slowing down the heart is useful in conditions such as atrial fibrillation, when the heart would otherwise beat much faster than normal. Slowing the heart increases diastolic filling time and allows the left ventricle to fill with more blood before contraction. This means stroke volume can be improved. This can help the modelling of the shape of the ventricle long-term. These effects on blood flow and contractility mean that digoxin can be useful even in patients who have a normal heart rate and are in sinus rhythm but who have heart failure.

NEGATIVE EFFECTS

Generally, patients tolerate digoxin well. However, the drug has a long half-life of 36 hours and if too much digoxin builds up in the body it can be toxic. About 80 % is excreted renally so patients with renal disease or patients who are elderly are more at risk of this. Digoxin toxicity is often difficult to recognise early on but symptoms include abdominal pain, nausea, vomiting, anorexia, tiredness, weakness, diarrhoea, changes in vision, changes in mood and confusion. The heart rate may be slowed excessively. As digoxin toxicity is often accompanied by hypokalaemia the patient is at risk of arrhythmia.

Toxicity can be detected by testing the blood for digoxin levels and is treated by stopping digoxin and treating complications if they arise. Any hypokalaemia should be corrected. Digibind, an injectable antidote, can be used in life-threatening cases but it is expensive and will not be carried as stock in all hospital pharmacies. The patient should be admitted for monitoring while the digoxin levels fall naturally after the drug is stopped.

EVIDENCE BASE

Digoxin is one of the oldest known medicines and in its plant form (digitalis or foxglove) has been used for centuries. Its modern use began in 1785 when Dr William Withering published a paper on its use in patients with 'dropsy', which we now call heart failure. The drug has been in and out of fashion since then and is used less in the United Kingdom than in other European countries.

A number of trials show the benefits of digoxin in patients with heart failure and atrial fibrillation (Wong & Rattery 2006). These benefits are in addition to standard treatment. Studies also look at whether digoxin is of use to heart failure patients who have sinus rhythm. In the RADIANCE (Packer et al. 1993) and PROVED trials (Uretsky et al. 1993) patients deteriorated if they were switched from digoxin to a placebo but the trials did not deal with the issue of mortality. Nor did the DIG trial find a mortality benefit, however the digoxin group required fewer hospitalisations than the placebo group for heart failure (Rich et al. 2001).

PRACTICAL CONSIDERATIONS

As digoxin has a long half-life a loading dose is necessary if the drug is used acutely to control a fast rhythm. If digoxin is introduced for a chronic condition no loading dose is needed. The long half-life means a once-a-day maintenance dose is possible.

Routine monitoring of digoxin levels is not recommended but can be measured if there are concerns about toxicity or compliance. Generally 1-2 nmol/l is therapeutic and >2 nmol/l is toxic. The digoxin plasma levels in the RADIANCE and PROVED trials did not affect treatment failure or changes to left ventricular ejection fraction so there is no definite evidence to recommend up-titration, although higher doses would be needed if the patient was still tachycardic. Higher serum levels did correlate with an increased risk of complications in those trials.

Other drugs that affect the electrolyte balance can affect digoxin levels, such as non-potassium-sparing diuretics, amphotericin B, corticosteroids, amiodarone, verapamil and nifidepine.

NITRATES

Vasodilator drugs can be very helpful for reducing breathlessness in patients with heart failure. In acute heart failure intravenous nitrates can be used while in chronic heart failure a small dose of long-acting nitrate and/or a short-acting nitrate, when required, can be useful.

Nitrates cause blood vessels to dilate directly. At lower doses they principally dilate the veins. This decreases venous return, reduces preload (left ventricular end diastolic pressure) and right-sided heart filling pressures and volume. At higher doses nitrates also act as arterial dilators, thereby lowering peripheral resistance, left ventricular pressures, myocardial work and oxygen demands. The final action is the one that is most well known – dilation of coronary arteries, thereby increasing blood and oxygen supply to the myocardium in order to relieve angina.

Short-acting nitrates can be useful in reducing exercise-induced and nocturnal breathlessness. Sublingual administration avoids first pass metabolism and leads to rapid action. They can also be used prophylactically before exertion. If a patient has less nocturnal breathlessness with a short-acting nitrate then a longer-acting nitrate at low dose, such as ISMN SR 30 mg, can also be tried.

The side-effects of nitrates are well understood. Some patients find they develop a headache rapidly after nitrate use, and some experience flushing and nausea. All these effects should be short-term. As the nitrate will lower blood pressure it is possible for a patient's blood pressure to drop so low that they are dizzy or even faint. This is more likely to happen if the patient already has a low blood pressure.

If nitrates are given continuously then their effectivesness decreases as the body becomes tolerant of them. This is due to the chemical depletion of a substance needed to turn the nitrates into nitrous oxide, the agent that acts on the smooth muscle walls to cause dilation. A nitrate-free period of 6 hours out of 24 hours is therefore recommended, and it is usually better to do this at night. However, some heart failure patients may find breathlessness harder to cope with at night and may prefer to have the nitrate-free period during the day.

OTHER VASODILATORS

Other vasodilators can also be considered for patients with heart failure. Hydralazine reduces the vascular resistance of arteries, reducing afterload and improving stroke volume. It has been used in combination with nitrates. Nitroprusside is an alpha-blocker that acts as a combined arterial and venous dilator, reducing filling pressures and improving stroke volume. Other drugs with vasodilating properties – such as verapamil and calcium channel blockers – have not been shown to be beneficial. Indeed, they are sometimes harmful for patients with heart failure, so they are not recommended for this type of use.

OXYGEN

If a patient is breathless a natural response is to assume they are short of oxygen. In fact this is rarely the case in patients with heart failure, unless they are acidotic or in acute heart failure with pulmonary oedema. Breathlessness is a complex sensation caused by a number of potential physiological mechanisms. Concurrent respiratory disease should also be considered.

If a patient with heart failure is hypoxic then supplementary oxygen can be helpful in improving symptoms. In the first instance, oxygen should be delivered via nasal cannula or mask until saturation is improved. But far more important for reducing acute breathlessness is treatment to attempt to eliminate the cause of the hypoxia – nitrates and diuretics to reduce preload and remove excess fluid, and nitrates and opiods to reduce afterload.

Oxygen should not be put on at a high flow rate without any effort to consider the underlying cause of the breathlessness or to establish oxygen saturation levels (ideally a full blood gas analysis). Unfortunately, this is occasionally still done in Accident and Emergency departments and by paramedics. The reason that it is not advisable is because it may not work and it may actually be harmful.

If a patient's blood has reached full saturation then no amount of extra oxygen is going to get into the blood as almost all oxygen is carried bound to haemoglobin cells, which have only a fixed number of receptors and once they are fully saturated, that is it. Only 3 % of oxygen is carried in the plasma and increasing this rate requires hyperbaric pressure in a special chamber. Excessive flow rates of oxygen therapy may be harmful in certain respiratory patients as this reduces their respiratory drive. Also, oxygen is a direct vasoconstricting agent so it could possibly make angina worse and raise blood pressure, which would worsen the patient's condition.

If the patient is chronically hypoxic then the use of oxygen is even more debatable as there is very little evidence that this is of any benefit in heart failure. Some patients do, however, feel better on oxygen. There may be a psychological element to this and the problem with this approach is that it limits the patient socially if they are dependent on oxygen being available. A working party of the Royal College of Physicians has recommended oxygen therapy for patients if their daytime hypoxaemia is $PaO_2 < 7.3\,kPa$ or nocturnal hypoxia is $SaO_2 < 90\,\%$ for at least 30 % of the night.

A particular circumstance where oxygen treatment might be of benefit is in patients with sleep apnoea, as this is associated with heart failure. In this case, nocturnal oxygen delivered through nasal cannula by a non-invasive intermittent positive pressure ventilator (NIPPV) or via a continuous positive airways pressure (CPAP) mask can be helpful and even remove sleep apnoea completely. However, the evidence base is limited as studies with heart failure patients have tended to be small and findings mixed. NICE does not make a firm recommendation for patients with heart failure.

INOTROPES

Inotropes are drugs that increase the contractility of the heart. Digoxin has a mildly positive inotropic effect and this was discussed earlier. Other inotropes that are sometimes used in patients with heart failure are those used intravenously in critical care settings during acute admission – principally dopamine and dobutamine for patients in cardiogenic shock.

Dopamine has several effects. It stimulates the beta-1 receptors to increase the force of contraction and stimulates alpha-receptors in the peripheral vascular system to cause vasoconstriction of those vessels. Dopamine receptors in the renal arteries are also stimulated to cause dilation. Dobutamine is more selective than dopamine and works mainly on the beta-receptors, although at high doses it can cause peripheral vasoconstriction.

There is only a weak evidence base for the positive effects of these agents in patients with heart failure but there is plenty of evidence that they can also cause harm – by increasing myocardial oxygen consumption, possibly increasing infarct size in patients with heart failure following acute myocardial infarction, provoking arrhythmias by increasing myocardial excitability, increasing heart rate and reducing diastolic coronary flow, as well as possibly constricting coronary arterioles (Elkayam et al. 2007; Shin et al. 2007). If inotropes are attempted they must be titrated carefully to avoid worsening the patient's condition.

Apart from the matter of careful dosing, inotropes require intravenous access through a central or long line. Ideally, central haemodynamic monitoring should also be used to guide their use. These issues tend to restrict their use to patients in critical care settings in acute hospitals.

ANTI-ARRHYTHMIC DRUGS

The high mortality rate due to arrhythmias in heart failure has led to an interest in whether anti-arrhythmic drugs are of any benefit. Unfortunately, such drugs in heart failure patients are associated with depression of left ventricular function and sometimes anti-arrhythmic drugs can also be pro-arrhythmic. Anti-arrhythmic drugs such as encainide, flecainide, moracizine, propafenone, verapamil and sotalol are thus best avoided in patients with heart failure.

The beta-blockers that are recommended for use in heart failure – bisoprolol and carvedilol – have anti-arrhythmic qualities and this is one of the key ways in which they reduce mortality in heart failure.

Studies show that the anti-arrhythmic drug amiodarone has a positive effect on mortality. It can be used in patients with heart failure as it is generally well-tolerated haemodynamically. In the GESICA study, patients had a left ventricular ejection fraction of around 20 % and were in NYHA class III or IV heart failure. They took amiodarone or a placebo. The results showed a mortality reduction of 28 % overall and a reduction in sudden death of 27 % in the group taking amiodarone (Doval et al. 1994).

Amiodarone is not without negative side-effects. Patients must be warned that while on the drug, excessive exposure to sunlight may turn their skin an orange-yellow colour. As amiodarone can also lead to thyroid and liver dysfunction, patients taking the drug should have blood tests to check these functions at least every six months.

OPIOIDS

Opioids have several possible roles in patients with heart failure. They can be very useful in stabilising patients with acute heart failure. They can also help to make severe breathlessness less of a burden. In end-stage heart failure, they are often important in the palliation of symptoms.

In acute heart failure, the left ventricle fails and afterload rises. Pressure rises in the chambers on the left side of the heart, while capillary hydrostatic pressure rises and fluid is forced out into the lung tissues, causing pulmonary oedema. As opioids have a venodilator effect they can reduce afterload. They also have the effect of making the patient feels calmer and dissociated from their body. As acute heart failure is very distressing, the patient feels out of control. Their adrenaline-mediated 'fight or flight' response becomes active, making the situation worse. By calming the patient down, time can be gained to allow other treatments, such as nitrates and diuretics, to take effect.

If severe chronic breathlessness has not responded to other treatments, it can be worth using opioids to attempt to reduce the effects of breathlessness. This approach has psychological and dependency issues so it is best reserved for patients who are highly disabled by their breathlessness and are struggling to cope. Opioids can be used occasionally to help prevent or relieve nocturnal breathlessness if this is a severe symptom.

The final role of opioids in heart failure is to treat patients who are reaching the end of their life. This is discussed in detail in Chapter 12.

DRUGS TO AVOID

There are several drugs that are best avoided for patients with heart failure. As this is not always possible, a risk analysis may be needed to establish if the benefits of using one of these drugs outweigh the potential risks. This is a decision that can alter over time and must be reviewed.

In the case of chemotherapy, the patient clearly does not have much choice. Sadly, it is fairly common for these patients to develop heart failure after chemotherapy, although it may not show for several years.

Box 10.16 Potentially Harmful Drugs in Heart Failure

Class	Examples	Reasons
NSAIDs	diclofenec, sodium and naproxen	Can cause fluid retention, hypertension and acute renal failure – double the renal risk if also taking diuretics.
Steroids	Prednisolone	Linked as a cause of heart failure. Can also lead to fluid retention.
Calcium channel blockers	Verapamil, diltiazem and nifedipine	Can cause fluid retention and also have a negative inotropic effect. Amlodipine is the safest to use in patients with heart failure.
Hypoglycaemic drugs	Rosiglitazone, pioglitazone and metformin	May lead to fluid retention. Metformin linked to lactic acidosis in renal failure.
Anti-arrhythmic drugs	Propafenone, sotalol and flecainide	Reduced contractility and can be pro-arrhythmic.
Tricyclic antidepressants	Amitryptyline	Reduced contractility and can be pro-arrhythmic.
Antifungal drugs	Itraconazole and amphotericin B	May reduce contractility and also be pro-arrhythmic.
Cytotoxic drugs	Anthracyclines, mitoxantrone, cyclophos-phamide, fluorouracil, capecitabine and trastuzumab	Disrupt myocardial cells and form free radicals leading to cardiomyopathy.

Box 10.17 Staged Treatment Algorithm for Chronic Heart Failure Medications

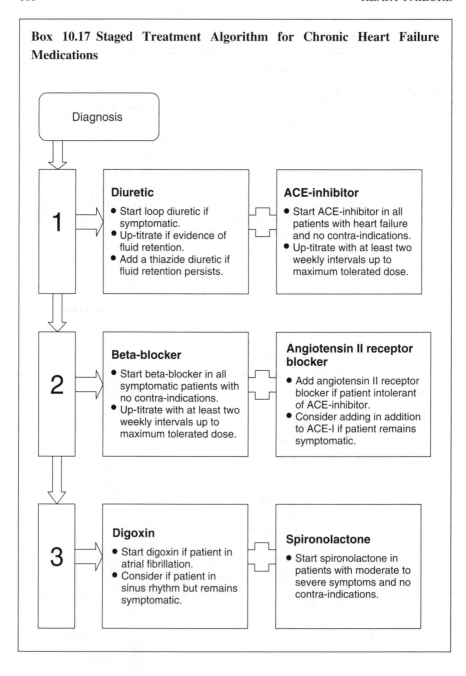

11 Invasive Treatments

This chapter outlines the various invasive procedures that can be used to treat heart failure – cardiac transplant, coronary revascularisation, cardiac assist devices, internal defibrillators and pacemakers. The indications, benefits, risks and evidence bases are discussed, along with how these procedures affect the patient and their nursing care.

ROLE OF INVASIVE TREATMENTS

We have seen how heart failure is chronic and incurable. In the early chapters the wide range of causes of heart failure and how they affect the structure and function of the heart were discussed. Invasive treatments can offer a range of benefits, such as stabilisation of the condition, symptom alleviation and improvements in function. Invasive treatments usually involve either surgical procedures or pacemaker devices. These procedures are carried out in tertiary cardiac centres. It is important for all staff to know something about them as an increasing number of patients is undergoing these procedures. These patients must be prepared for the procedure and cared for post-procedure – roles that can devolve to all staff in contact with the patient. It is important to understand the potential benefits, limitations and side-effects of these procedures.

Box 11.1 Summary of Invasive Interventions

Cardiac surgery

Cardiac transplant	For patients with severe heart failure but without end-organ damage or significant other co-morbidities.
Coronary revascularisation	For patients with ischaemic cardiomyopathy and evidence of ongoing reversible ischaemia.
Cardiac valve surgery	For patients whose heart failure is caused by an operable valve disorder.

Box 11.1 (Continued)

Left ventricle reduction	For patients whose heart failure is being exacerbated by a dilated or aneurysmal left ventricle.

Devices

Biventricular pacemakers	For patients with severe heart failure, dysynchronicity and an intraventricular conduction delay.
Internal cardiac defibrillators	For patients with a higher risk of life-threatening arrhythmias.
Cardiac assist devices	For patients with severe heart failure as a bridge to transplant, bridge to recovery or destination therapy.
Intra-aortic balloon pumps	Temporary measure for patients with acute severe heart failure as a bridge to transplant or recovery.

CARDIAC SURGERY

Surgery can replace or repair a damaged heart. A cardiac transplant replaces a damaged and failing heart and is a highly specialised and complex operation performed on adults at six specialist centres in the United Kingdom – in Birmingham, Glasgow, South Manchester, Harefield, Papworth and Newcastle. In patients with particular problems that are causing or contributing to their heart failure, such as coronary artery disease or valve disease, operations can repair or stabilise the damage. Coronary artery bypass grafting (CABG) and cardiac valve repair or replacement are performed routinely in tertiary sector regional cardiac units. There is also a range of experimental or less common surgical procedures sometimes undertaken to change the shape of the ventricle in heart failure.

Patients with heart failure can undergo surgery and do so regularly. However, their operative risk is always likely to be greater than someone without heart failure because of their impaired haemodynamics, the risk of neurohormonal pathological responses to operative stresses, and the increased risk of arrhythmias. Surgeons have scoring systems to enable them to calculate actual operative risks for individuals undergoing various types of surgery. Some surgeons and anaesthetists will be willing to take on higher risk patients and others will not. Patients with heart failure are a diverse group; some heart failure patients may be operable and others not. The other consideration is the nature of the proposed surgery. Some surgery is life saving or crucial for functioning and, in these cases, the benefit may outweigh the risk. Other surgeries may have less clear benefits and the outcomes may seem limited or not realistic.

CARDIAC TRANSPLANT

If the heart is not working properly and is deteriorating then a logical response is to think about replacing the heart. Sometimes patients themselves will ask if they can have a 'new' heart.

The technique of a cardiac transplant was developed from the 1960s by the South African surgeon, Christian Barnard, who carried out the first human cardiac transplant. The procedure involves removing the patient's own heart and replacing it with a donor heart. The donor heart has to be used almost immediately so two surgical teams are needed, requiring precise co-ordination. Before the transplant, patients must be selected carefully for suitability and post procedure, the patient is committed to a life-long regime of anti-rejection drugs.

There are no randomised controlled trials of cardiac transplantation and heart failure, due to the inherent research difficulties, but there have been observational studies. These show an improved quality of life after a transplant and a 70-80 % survival rate at five years (UK Transplant 2007). The long-term prognosis is affected by the side-effects of immunosupression treatment (renal failure, infection, malignancy and hypertension) and the development of graft vascular disease. There are no recent health economic data from the United Kingdom on cardiac transplants: although it is an expensive procedure, the benefits for the individual patient can be enormous.

Not all patients are suitable for a cardiac transplant. The patient must have severe enough heart failure to justify the risks of the procedure. At the same time, they have to be physically and psychologically fit enough for the operation and the long-term monitoring and treatment post operation.

The initial referral for a cardiac transplant consideration at a regional transplant centre is made by the patient's cardiologist. The NICE guidelines recommend that referral for a transplant assessment should be considered for patients with severe refractory symptoms or cardiogenic shock (NICE 2003). Patients would be contra-indicated if they are drug or alcohol abusers or if they have any of the following: an uncontrolled mental illness, cancer within the past five years, a systematic disease with multi-organ involvement, an uncontrolled infection, severe renal failure (in some centres), high pulmonary vascular resistance, recent thromboembolitic complications, an active peptic ulcer, severe liver impairment, or other diseases with a poor prognosis. Outcomes tend to be better with younger patients and so most centres have an upper age limit (usually 65 years old) for accepting patients for a cardiac transplant. The patient sees the team at the transplant centre for various investigations and assessments. If the patient is accepted and wishes to go forward with a transplant, then they will go on to the transplant waiting list. Patients must have a donor heart matched to their blood group and body size.

Box 11.2 Suitability for Cardiac Transplant

Indications	Contra-indications
• severe symptoms (NYHA class IV) • on full medical therapy • cardiogenic shock.	• significant co-morbidity (see text) • drug or alcohol misuse • non-concordant with treatments • uncontrolled mental illness

---

In the United Kingdom at present there are only about 200–300 cardiac transplants per year (UK Transplant 2007). This number has actually decreased from a few years ago. This is a reflection of the reduced availability of donor hearts, probably due to changes in road traffic accident fatalities. As there are around one million patients with heart failure in the United Kingdom, the scale of the problem is immediately apparent: the number of patients who will receive a cardiac transplant is overwhelmingly short of those who could benefit from one. This places even more of an emphasis on targeting the donor hearts towards those whose need is greatest. A cardiac transplant replaces the whole heart – yet for upwards of 90 % of patients it could be argued that left ventricular support is the priority and treatments such as left ventricular assist devices could be used more widely.

Some patients view cardiac transplants as a panacea but the reality is more complex. It can be a struggle psychologically for some patients to cope with a donor organ, perhaps the heart especially because of its socio-cultural connotations. Some patients have difficulty with the drug regimes. Patients may also find that their improvement post operation is not as significant as they had hoped and that rehabilitation is a long process. It is worth remembering that a transplant does not necessarily change the underlying disease processes.

CORONARY REVASCULARISATION

In Chapter 3 we noted that in the United Kingdom around two-thirds of heart failure is as a result of coronary heart disease. Myocardial infarction can leave viable but ischaemic myocardium – also known as 'hibernating' myocardium – where the cells have enough blood supply to survive but not enough to work normally. Ischaemic myocardium can be a source of arrhythmias. Infarcted tissue never recovers full contractility on its own and over time remodelling of the myocardium occurs. With revascularisation, arrhythmias can be reduced (with an impact on mortality), contractility improved and the left ventricular ejection fraction increased. For this to work there has to be a sufficiently viable myocardium. Reversibility of ischaemia can be judged subjectively by whether the patient's angina responds to nitrates and objectively by stress echocardiography and angiography. If the ischaemia is irreversible then there is no point in revascularisation.

Coronary revascularisation can take place either through coronary artery bypass grafting (CABG) or through percutaneous coronary intervention (PCI). The outcomes are argued fiercely – with strong advocates for the superiority of both techniques and the results being difficult to interpret due to emerging techniques making older data less relevant – but tend to be broadly similar (Morrison 2006). The coronary artery bypass graft is a more invasive and complex procedure involving a general anaesthetic, usually a heart and lung circulatory bypass, intensive care and a typical inpatient stay of 5–10 days. Severe left ventricular dysfunction increases the operative risks for coronary artery bypass grafting. However, a poorer left ventricular ejection fraction means that there are better potential symptom improvements, although not long-term survival benefits, if the patient survives the operation (Pocar et al. 2007). In contrast, a percutaneous coronary intervention is done under local anaesthesia as a day case procedure and has a lower risk profile.

Coronary revascularisation does not bring benefits to all patients and it is wise to be cautious about potential benefits for complex symptoms such as breathlessness. The benefits of revascularisation for patients with heart failure tend to be supported by studies of patients with moderate to severe left ventricular systolic dysfunction. There are no specific randomised controlled trials looking at revascularisation as a treatment for heart failure but there are the findings of cohort studies and subgroup analyses of patients with heart failure recruited for revascularisation trials. There are no clear data on the cost effectiveness of revascularisation in heart failure. The NICE guidelines' recommendation is that revascularisation should not routinely be considered in patients with left ventricular impairment unless they have ongoing angina (NICE 2003).

CARDIAC VALVE SURGERY

Some patients have heart failure as a result of a diseased cardiac valve. A tight, stenotic valve can lead to a rise in chamber pressure as a compensatory mechanism and this can lead to hypertrophy. A leaking, regurgitant valve will lead to an excess chamber volume which can lead to dilation. When the valve is diseased, surgical repair or replacement of the valve may relieve the heart failure.

Not all patients with failing valves and heart failure will be suitable for valve surgery. The progression may be that the patient first had heart failure and the valve is now failing as a result of changes to the shape of the heart from the heart failure. For example, as the left ventricle fails it dilates and the mitral valve leaflets fail to meet, leading to a central jet of mitral regurgitation into the left atrium. In this case, surgery on the valve is unlikely to be successful or to endure.

Sometimes in patients with ischaemia and heart failure the mitral valve may also be failing and some surgeons perform repairs to or replacement of the mitral valve alongside coronary artery bypass grafting.

Cardiac valves will be replaced either with tissue valves or artificial valves. Tissue valves have a shorter lifespan than artificial valves but do not require anti-coagulation – for these reasons they are preferred in older patients. Patients who have cardiac valves replaced with artificial valves will need life-long anticoagulation, usually with warfarin, due to the increased thrombotic risk. Patients with valve replacements need regular follow-ups and periodic echocardiograms to check their valve.

LEFT VENTRICLE REDUCTION

Various surgical operations can change the shape of the heart. For patients with large left ventricular aneurysms there is an aneurysmectomy. This is a surgical reversal of myocardial remodelling. A section of the left ventricle is cut out and the remainder patched and resewn to reshape the cavity from globular to elliptical, without reducing cavity volume, in order to improve function. This is also known as the Dor procedure. There is also the option of surgically reducing the size of the ventricle through overlapping cardiac volume reduction (OLCVR) surgery with papillary muscle plication (PMP) (Matsui et al. 2005).

DEVICES

A number of cardiological devices have been developed to help patients with heart conditions. Many of these have applications for patients with heart failure. These devices tend to be inserted by cardiologists rather than cardiac surgeons.

PACEMAKERS

A pacemaker consists of a processor/battery box and wire(s) that sense and pace the heart. The box is usually implanted in a pectoral muscle pocket on the left side of the upper chest and the wire is threaded through the subclavian vein to the right side of the heart – usually the endocardial wall of the right ventricle, but sometimes also the right atrium for a dual chamber model. A pacemaker is fitted under local anaesthetic and is a day case or overnight stay depending on local policy. The length of the procedure varies depending on the technical complexity of the patient's anatomy and what type of system is being implanted.

Standard pacemakers are used predominately in patients with conduction disorders, such as sick sinus syndrome and heart blocks. Sometimes patients with fast atrial flutter/fibrillation or other supraventricular tachycardias are also paced after HIS ablation. Traditional right-sided dual chamber pacemakers have never shown great benefits for patients with heart failure except where there was an atrioventricular (AV) node delay of more than 100 ms. Such a delay indicates a dyssynchronicity between the left and right sides of the heart.

Dyssynchronicity is common in heart failure and it is logical that a heart that is less co-ordinated will be less efficient and have to work harder to produce cardiac output. In recent years a new technique has been developed to pace both the left and right sides of the heart to return the heart to normal synchronicity – known as biventricular pacing or cardiac resynchronisation therapy (CRT). This is done in the same manner as for a dual chamber pacemaker except that a third wire is threaded through the coronary sinus at the back of the heart to enable left ventricle pacing. By pacing both sides of the heart a more normal physiological pacing is possible.

In around 30 % of patients with heart failure the enlargement of the heart, or previous infarctions, can cause an intraventricular septal conduction delay, such as left or right bundle branch block with a QRS > 120 ms (Chow et al. 2003). Having a conduction disorder seems to be both a symptom of worsening heart failure and a contributing cause. Cardiac resynchronisation improves cardiac function and output, symptoms and exercise tolerance and reduces hospitalisations. Biventricular pacemakers are cost effective (Feldman et al. 2005; Calvert et al. 2005; Yao et al. 2007). Although the devices cost more than a standard pacemaker and the procedure is more complex technically, with more time in the cardiac catheter laboratory as a result, the lower rehospitalisation rates make them a very effective therapy.

Box 11.3 Evidence Base for Biventricular Pacemakers in Heart Failure

MUSTIC (Linde et al. 2003)	MUSTIC involved only 68 patients but found that exercise capacity and functional status were improved significantly, as were quality of life, peak oxygen uptake and ejection fraction in patients that had a biventricular pacemaker.
MIRACLE (Young et al. 2003)	MIRACLE showed significant improvements in quality of life, exercise tolerance, NYHA class, peak oxygen uptake and ejection fraction in patients who received a biventricular pacemaker. It also reported lower heart failure admissions in the biventricular pacemaker group.
COMPANION-CHF (Saxon et al. 2006)	COMPANION was halted early because of a 20 % reduction in mortality and rehospitalisation in the biventricular pacing group. In the arm that had a biventricular pacemaker and internal defibrillator the mortality reduction was 40 %.
CARE-HF (Cleland et al. 2005)	CRT significantly reduced mortality (36 %, $P < 0.002$) in patients with NYHA functional class III and class IV heart failure and ventricular dyssynchrony. This study also showed that CRT reverses ventricular remodelling and improves myocardial performance progressively for at least 18 months.

For patients to be considered suitable for cardiac resynchronisation therapy they must have moderate to severe symptoms (intractable despite optimal medical therapy), systolic dysfunction, no significant mitral regurgitation and have a QRS complex of > 120 ms. Even with these preconditions cardiac resynchronisation is ineffective in about a third of patients who have biventricular pacemakers (Rosanio et al. 2005). The reasons for this are not clear. It is likely that there will be improvements to this figure as the technology develops and more is discovered about which patients are likely to benefit in advance of implantations.

Many other questions remain about cardiac resynchronisation therapy: is right-sided pacing needed or is left ventricle pacing enough? Which population benefits most? Are QRS delays of more than 150 ms needed to show signs of improvement? What is the optimal position to pace the left ventricle? Some of these areas are very unclear – a recent follow-up study of patients after cardiac resynchronisation therapy actually found patients who had a QRS < 120 ms had better outcomes (with similar baseline characteristics) than those who had a wider QRS (Gasparini et al. 2007).

It is important also to bear in mind that patients can have problems peri- and post-procedure. There can be technical difficulties in inserting a biventricular pacemaker, such as difficult anatomy and phrenic nerve stimulation. Like all pacemakers, they require regular follow-ups to check settings and battery life. At the end of the battery life the battery will need to be changed. When the patient dies the pacemakers will need to be removed, especially before cremation, to avoid a battery explosion.

Box 11.4 NICE Recommendation on Biventricular Pacemakers

NICE recommends that cardiac resynchronisation should be considered in patients with left ventricular systolic dysfunction (left ventricular ejection fraction < 35 %), drug refractory symptoms and QRS > 120 ms.

INTERNAL CARDIAC DEFIBRILLATORS (ICD)

Patients with heart failure and who do not die of non-cardiac causes will die of either pump failure or a sudden arrhythmic death. With medication, more patients are surviving for longer and having greater exposure to life-threatening ventricular arrhythmias, which are common in heart failure. Up to half of patients with heart failure now die of an arrhythmia (Goldstein 2004). The usual medical treatment for arrhythmias are class I and class III anti-arrhythmic drugs but these are problematic in heart failure and only amiodarone is considered reasonably safe to use in patients with heart failure (Piepoli et al. 1998b). Even with full concordance of optimal medications the risk of arrhythmia recurrence is 40–50 % at five years.

Since the 1960s, life-threatening arrhythmias have been treated with an electrical cardioversion in hospitals either as an emergency or an elective procedure. From the 1970s, the concept of having an automated internal cardiac defibrillator implanted in high risk patients, ready to defibrillate if a life-threatening arrhythmia occurred, was developed and they were first implanted in humans in the 1980s. The first generation of internal cardiac defibrillators was large and had to be sited in the abdomen with thoracotomies for the electrode positioning. Further device generations have reduced in size to little bigger than standard pacemakers, with a similar percutaneous implantation and pectoral position for the battery box. Improvements in technology have also improved functionality with anti-tachycardic pacing, low-energy synchronised cardioversion and high-energy (up to 30 J) defibrillation. Energy levels are a lot lower than for external defibrillation because there is no thoracic impedance to the energy when it is delivered directly to the heart.

Internal cardiac defibrillators are implanted under a local anaesthetic and sedation. A 5–8 cm incision is made in the left intraclavicular region with either a subcutaneous or deep pectoral pocket made for the battery box to sit in. Leads are inserted: a ventricular lead for sensing, pacing and defibrillation; an atrial lead for dual chamber pacing; and the option of a third left ventricular lead for biventricular pacing. The leads are connected to the battery box, pacing checks are made for sensing and ventricular fibrillation is induced to check the defibrillation option. Post-procedure care is similar to that of pacemakers, with a discharge within 24–48 hours and regular outpatient follow-ups. If the defibrillator is used then the device should be interrogated afterwards. Battery life has improved – depending on how often they are used, current batteries are expected to last 7–9 years.

Patients with internal cardiac defibrillators are allowed to drive once the device has been in for six months or more and if it has not delivered a shock for at least six months. If the device is implanted for primary prevention then the patient needs only to stop driving for one month post procedure. Licences are reviewed annually; however, Public Service Vehicle and Heavy Goods Vehicle drivers are permanently disqualified. Further details can be found at the DVLA website.

The first set of problems encountered with internal cardiac defibrillators are similar to those in patients with a pacemaker: infection, erosion, conductor/insulator fracture and over- and under-sensing. The unique complication that can occur with internal cardiac defibrillators is inappropriate shocks. This usually occurs with fast atrial fibrillation but may also occur with very fast sinus tachycardia. Devices are becoming more sophisticated and either the parameters can be reprogrammed to be less sensitive or further anti-arrhythmic medication can be given to control the rate in atrial arrhythmias or sinus tachycardia. Occasionally it may be necessary in uncontrolled atrial fibrillation to ablate the atrioventricular node and pace the patient alongside the internal cardiac defibrillator.

Experiencing a shock is unpleasant for the patient and distressing for family members who are present. It is difficult to fully prepare the patient for a shock and some patients find the experience, or the uncertainty of when the next shock might happen, very difficult to cope with psychologically. Then again, other patients adapt well and see the defibrillator as a life-enhancing device which reduces their worry.

Although many patients with heart failure have arrhythmias, not all of them do. A question then arises as to which heart failure patients should have internal cardiac defibrillators. They are definitely indicated as a secondary prevention for those patients who have survived ventricular fibrillation or ventricular tachycardia arrests. A large systematic review showed that internal cardiac defibrillators prolong life in patients with impaired left ventricular function and a history of ventricular arrhythmias. In a meta analysis of the AVID, CIDS and CASH trials there was a 28 % mortality reduction in those given an internal cardiac defibrillator over those treated with amiodarone alone. This was as true for ventricular tachycardia as it was for ventricular fibrillation as the background arrhythmia. A subgroup analysis showed that those patients with a left ventricular ejection fraction < 35 % had an even greater mortality benefit of 34 % with an internal cardiac defibrillator compared with patients treated with amiodarone alone (Connolly et al. 2000a).

There is also evidence that ICDs should be used as a primary prevention in patients with evidence of previous ventricular arrhythmias on ECGs and in patients with low ejection fractions, regardless of whether the patients have had a ventricular arrhythmia cardiac arrest. Patients with advanced heart failure and internal cardiac defibrillators have a better survival rate but a shorter time to rehospitalisation than those without (Nazarian et al. 2005).

Box 11.5 Trials of Internal Cardiac Defibrillators

AVID (The AVID Investigators 1997).	In the AVID (Antiarrhythmics vs. Implantable Defibrillator) study 1013 patients were followed up for 3 years. Relative mortality reduction was 27–39 % $(+/-20)$ in the ICD group. It concluded that among survivors of ventricular fibrillation or sustained ventricular tachycardia causing severe symptoms, ICDs were superior to anti-arrhythmic drugs for increasing overall survival.
CIDS (Connolly et al 2000b)	In the CIDS (Canadian Implantable Defibrillator) study 659 patients with resuscitated VF or VT or with unmonitored syncope had ICD or amiodarone. It found a 20 % relative risk reduction occurred in all-cause mortality and a 33 % reduction occurred in arrhythmic mortality with ICD therapy compared with amiodarone, but this reduction did not reach statistical significance.
CASH (Kuck et al. 2000)	In the CASH (Cardiac Arrest Study Hamburg) study patients had an ICD or one of a selection of anti-arrhythmic drugs and were followed up for an average of 57 months. It found a 23 % reduction in all-cause mortality in the ICD group but this reduction did not reach statistical significance.
MADIT-II (Moss et al. 2002)	In the MADIT-II study patients who had had a prior MI and advanced heart failure had an ICD or anti-arrhythmic drugs. In the ICD group there was a 31 % reduction in mortality over an average 20-month follow-up.

Box 11.5 (Continued)

MUSTT (Buxton et al. 1999)	In the MUSTT study 704 patients, with a history of MI, poor ejection fraction and VT on ECG, received an ICD, or anti-arrhythmic drugs, or neither. Five-year mortality in the ICD group was 24 %, whereas it was 48 % for the non-treated group and slightly worse in the drug group.
SCD-HeFT (Bardy et al. 2005)	The SCD-HEFT study involved 2521 patients and compared amiodarone with implantable defibrillators in heart failure patients. There was an absolute reduction of all-cause mortality of 7 % in the ICD group over five years. No significant mortality benefit was observed in the amiodarone arm compared with the placebo group.

In the United Kingdom the implantation rate for internal cardiac defibrillators has been significantly lower, at around 17 per million population per year, than in the United States and most of Western Europe (NICE 2003). This has largely been due to financial reasons as the devices cost £20 000 and, until recently, individual health authority agreements to fund the device had to be sought for each patient. A relative lack of specialist cardiologists (electrophysiologists) has also put a brake on implantation. Now that the arrhythmia chapter of the *National Service Framework for Coronary Heart Disease* has been published there is more attention being paid to and funding for these devices and many more are being implanted.

As a greater number of internal defibrillators are inserted some questions about their use are likely to become more prominent. They have been shown to increase longevity but the patient will, of course, still die at some stage. The difference is that the balance of the causes of death will change, with fewer sudden arrhythmic deaths and more slower circulatory deaths. Another issue that is likely to become more evident is dealing with internal defibrillators at the end of a patient's life. A patient who is at the end stage of heart failure will need to have their defibrillator deactivated, otherwise it may well shock as patients frequently have ventricular arrhythmias as they die. There is a question mark over who is going to deactivate these devices as they become more prevalent. At the present time it is largely done by technicians from the tertiary centres going out to patients. This may not be a sustainable model in the future.

Box 11.6 Indications for Internal Cardiac Defibrillator Insertion

- primary prevention – in patients with LVEF < 35 % and non-sustained VT
- secondary prevention – in patients who have survived VT/VF cardiac arrests

CARDIAC ASSIST DEVICES

There has been interest for many years in supporting or replacing the failing heart with artificial pumps. Complete artificial hearts have been developed but are still experimental, whereas left ventricular assist devices (LVADs) are being seen more in clinical practice – particularly in the United States – with different models available. These artificial heart pumps boost the performance of the failing left ventricle.

They arose from work in the 1960s by Dr Debakey and have been further developed to the present day (Frazier 2003). Models can involve the pump being inserted either inside or outside of the ventricle. The latest models are thumb sized, silent and can pump up to six litres of blood per minute. The pump fits in the failing ventricle and is connected percutaneously to a controller and battery pack about the size of a mobile telephone.

The benefit of a left ventricular assist device is the maintenance of a reasonable cardiac output in patients with severe heart failure. A left ventricular assist device can be used in one of three ways: as a bridge to cardiac transplant, as a bridge to recovery and as destination therapy. The most common indication has been to keep a severely ill and deteriorating patient alive until undergoing a cardiac transplant. The device can prevent death while the patient waits for a transplant and improve outcomes after the transplant (Frazier 2003). They are now also used as a short-term bridge to recovery because the improved cardiac output can improve organ dysfunction, while the reduction in congestion improves left ventricle remodelling. They are most useful in patients who have developed acute severe heart failure – such as with myocarditis – and do not have significant co-morbidity. The improved mortality in heart failure patients who had left ventricular assist devices as destination therapy was shown in the REMATCH trial (Rose et al. 2001). It is worth noting that left ventricular assist devices have been trialled only with systolic dysfunction and not diastolic dysfunction (Jessup & Brozena 2003).

As a destination therapy, left ventricular assist devices have been used less, as there remain issues around tolerability and longevity of battery life. The problems with left ventricular assist devices have tended to be technical and clinical. Size and noise were an issue in early models. All models at present still require an external power source. This means that batteries must be changed and spares carried. It also means there is a potential infection risk.

Cardiac support devices have several advantages over cardiac transplants. The most obvious is that they are potentially far more available than donor hearts. The second advantage is that they do not involve ethical issues to the extent of cardiac transplants. Finally, as device costs decrease, they become a much more cost-effective option than cardiac transplants. A Health Technology Assessment study considered the clinical and cost effectiveness of left ventricular assist devices (Clegg et al. 2005). The study found that while left ventricular assist devices appear to be effective in improving the survival rate of patients with end-stage heart failure, more work is needed on the methodological quality and strength of the evidence to support this.

INTRA-AORTIC BALLOON PUMPS (IABP)

Intra-aortic balloon pumps are mechanical devices used temporarily to support circulation in critical care hospital areas. They were first used in 1968 by Krantrowitz and colleagues (Krantrowitz et al. 1968) and developed in the 1970s.

A long sausage-like catheter is inserted up the femoral artery into the aorta. This is connected to a machine that then inflates the tube in time with diastole in the cardiac cycle – known as *counter-pulsation*. By doing so, it is hoped to increase diastolic blood pressure, augment coronary blood flow and reduce ventricular afterload.

Intra-aortic balloon pumps are used post surgery and sometimes as bridges to recovery in patients immediately after myocardial infarctions or with acute severe heart failure with a recoverable cause, such as myocarditis. Balloon pumps can be effective but as the patient's haemodynamics improve only by 15 % at best this may not be adequate for the recovery of all patients (Oshima et al. 2005). As a stabilisation measure there is some evidence they help to decrease mortality (Visser & Purday 1998). However, they are a short-term measure as the patient is bed-bound and at increased risk of a thrombosis and infections.

EMERGING TECHNOLOGIES

Over the past ten years, emerging technologies that offer the prospect of a cure for heart failure have generated much interest and media attention. The first of these was gene therapy, which has since been overtaken in the headlines by stem cell therapy. Although these treatments are still at an experimental stage rather than being available clinically to heart failure patients, due to their high media profile, patients often ask about them.

GENE THERAPY

Gene therapies offer the potential for treatment of heart failure in a number of ways (Pachori et al. 2006). In animal studies, gene injection into the aortic root or by intracoronary injection has improved systolic and diastolic function, contractility and left ventricular function, and had a positive effect on ventricular remodelling (Hambleton et al. 2006). The mechanisms of action are thought to include effects on calcium in the myocytes and beta-adrenaline signalling down-regulation.

As the results from the initial animal studies were so promising, gene therapy was perhaps over-hyped at first, with the claims rushing ahead of the science (French 1998). The applicability of the therapy to humans is not straightforward (Sesti & Kloner 2004). Gene transfer up until now has involved the use of viral vectors but these have the disadvantage of causing an immunological response. It is not known at this point if improvements in left ventricular function are long-term.

STEM CELL THERAPY

Human tissue has a greater or lesser ability to regenerate itself when damaged. In degenerative diseases, such as diabetes or Parkinson's disease, the cells are not normally replaced or repaired once damaged. In the heart, there is a natural process whereby the heart tries to achieve some regeneration. For example, when the myocardium is under–perfused, growth factors are released in order to stimulate angiogenesis – the formation of new blood vessels – which can be seen as small collateral coronary vessels on angiography. This natural process is, however, limited and there is a great deal of research interest in ways to stimulate this process through clinical intervention.

One of the most promising treatments involves the injection of stem cells. These are cells which the body uses as part of self-renewal and which have the potential to develop and specialise in different ways depending on where they are placed. Stem cells can be harvested in adults from bone marrow or from the heart itself. The problem with adult stem cell collection is that the range of cells available is limited. In embryos, there are large cores of undifferentiated stem cells that can develop into any cells. Hence the interest in using these embryonic cells for cellular therapy in regenerative medicine. There are a number of ethical concerns regarding using embryos in this way and to date their use is prohibited or limited in most countries (Gerecht & Itskovitz 2004).

Once collected and processed, stem cells can be injected using either an intracoronary method or injecting directly into the endocardial wall (Widimsky et al. 2006; Bartenek et al. 2007). Studies of animal models of bone marrow cells show they have the potential to improve myocardial perfusion and function in ischaemic heart disease, reverse remodelling and regenerate myocardium and coronary capillaries (Perin et al. 2003; Patel et al. 2005; Lipiecki et al. 2006; Shepler & Patel 2007). Small trials in humans have begun and have shown benefits such as myocyte regeneration in myocardial infarction and ischaemic cardiomyopathy, with reductions in infarct size and improvements in the ejection fraction, myocardial perfusion and wall motion (Dawn et al. 2005).

The results to date are promising and bone marrow stem cell therapy into the heart appears safe, but the number of trials and patients, along with the length of follow-up, remain small. More research is needed and a lot of questions need to be answered before stem cell therapy becomes a routine heart failure treatment (Bartenek et al. 2007; Collins et al. 2007). In theory, stem cell treatment offers a range of benefits, from an alternative to cardiac transplant to a reversal of existing damage in all patients with evidence of heart failure. However, most of the trials thus far look at stem cell treatment in the context of acute myocardial infarction, while their role in chronic heart failure remains less clear (Allan et al. 2007).

12 End-Stage Heart Failure

In this chapter, end of life issues for patients with heart failure are discussed. The difficulties of predicting prognosis, talking about end of life issues with patients and providing a dignified death at the end of a patient's life are considered. The role of specialist palliative care services and the contributions of other members of the wider multi-disciplinary team are debated.

DEFINING 'END-STAGE' HEART FAILURE

Most clinicians who see patients with heart failure have an idea of what they mean when they describe a patient as having end-stage heart failure. Their experience tells them that the severity of that patient's heart failure means the patient's prognosis is poor. Whilst the subjective 'gut feeling' of an expert is very valuable it can be more difficult to define objectively why a patient is coming to the end of their life. There are some markers which research shows are usually related to end-stage heart failure – see Box 12.1

Box 12.1 Markers for End Stage Heart Failure

- severe symptoms of heart failure at rest (NYHA class IV)
- evidence of rapidly worsening end-organ damage (renal or liver failure, confusion)
- poor left ventricular ejection fraction
- no further heart failure treatment options available

Many people have contemplated ways of finding markers for poor prognosis in individual patients. The two factors that consistently emerge from studies are that poor prognosis is predicted by the frequency of re-admissions to hospital and rapidly worsening renal function (Khan et al. 2005). This makes sense as a patient who is repeatedly admitted to hospital for heart failure has heart failure that is poorly controlled or becoming unresponsive to treatment, while if the kidney function is declining rapidly due to heart failure then renal perfusion must be very poor. A poor ejection fraction and raised BNP are also markers of a poor prognosis as they indicate severe disease. Symptoms and functional class are less predictive – some patients have severe symptoms or functional disability but are in fact stable at that level – but symptoms at rest are a sign of a poor prognosis. The prognosis will also vary between the sexes, ages, types of heart failure and what co-morbidities the patient has.

Unlike cancer, heart failure patients do not have a tipping point where they suddenly get worse. Rather, they have a series of deteriorations from which they recover partially until either the patient dies of sudden death or goes into cardiogenic shock. This makes recognising the point at which they are actively dying difficult compared with cancer disease progression.

Box 12.2 Disease Progression

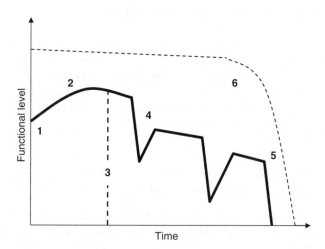

(1) Patients with heart failure often have many symptoms and poor functional level on diagnosis.
(2) They may improve functionally with optimised treatment.
(3) Sudden death is possible at any point.
(4) Patients will be acutely unwell when decompensated but can rally, often not getting quite back to how they were.
(5) Functional level continues to deteriorate as the heart fails, acute decompensation becomes more frequent and eventually the heart does not rally.
(6) In contrast, patients with cancer often start with a better functional level then reach a point where they have a sudden deterioration towards death.

The progression of the disease is problematic in that it is difficult to know when to start discussing end of life issues in more detail with a patient and to start making referrals and setting up services for the end of life. It is very common for heart failure patients to deteriorate severely and be thought near to death only to rally and recover some function. This may mean that palliative services have to be put in place and then removed. The progression may also be more gradual in heart failure than in cancer. All of these variations mean that end of life care in heart failure patients may need to be different in some respects compared with patients dying of cancer. For example, the Gold Standards Framework 'surprise' test (i.e. 'Would you be surprised if this patient died in the next 12 months?' – If no, treat as palliative care) if applied to heart failure patients would mean most of them being considered for palliative care. The approach is right, however, – to use clinical judgement.

THE DYING HEART

It is possible to observe two broad patterns in the dying heart. The first pattern is sudden death, which can occur at any point but the risks are higher as heart failure progresses, and the second pattern is that of heart failure with failure to compensate, leading to cardiogenic shock.

Sudden cardiac death is usually caused by fast arrhythmias. The usual life-threatening tachyarrhythmias are ventricular tachycardia and ventricular fibrillation. This can occur in anyone at any time but we have seen that life-threatening arrhythmias are much more common in heart failure. This is thought to be due to a number of possible mechanisms – see Box 12.3. Fast arrhythmias are also much less likely to be tolerated by a weak heart. Unless reversed, there will be a rapid drop in cardiac output and the patient will lose consciousness and die in a short space of time. Sudden cardiac death is thought to be the cause of around half of the deaths in heart failure.

Box 12.3 Causes of Arrhythmias in Heart Failure

- high circulating catecholamine (e.g. beta-adrenaline)
- electrolyte disturbances
- disruption of electrical pathways in heart (such as scarring post infarction)
- structural changes and dyssynchronicity
- pressure of volume overload of the cardiac chambers

It is, of course, feasible to resuscitate someone with a life-threatening arrhythmia by defibrillating the heart (resetting the polarity so it reverts to a co-ordinated rhythm). For this to work – and it works in only about 20 % of cases in hospital – defibrillation must be undertaken very quickly as brain injury occurs after only a couple of minutes (Gwinnutt et al. 2000). We saw in Chapter 11 how internal defibrillators reduce the risk of sudden cardiac death and how heart failure patients in particular are benefiting from these devices. Having an internal defibrillator does not, of course, prevent the patient from dying. If a patient does not die of an arrhythmia then they will die, hopefully much later, of end-stage heart failure.

Dying of end-stage heart failure means that the patient will have a progressively worse cardiac output as the heart fails to compensate to maintain cardiac output. Failure to compensate is a combination of the effects of cardiac remodelling and myocyte changes leading to poor contractility, cardiac dilatation leading to Laplace's Law taking effect plus increasingly ineffective neurohormonal regulation. This failure to compensate produces a worsening of the patient's symptoms and the dropping cardiac output will itself lead to further symptoms. In these circumstances, a palliative care approach is mandatory: relieving symptoms as far as possible, removing treatments that are no longer of benefit, and reducing suffering through physical, psychological and spiritual support.

At this stage the patient is moving into cardiogenic shock – the inability of the heart to deliver sufficient blood to meet resting tissue metabolic demands (Barry & Sarembock 1998). The patient will develop metabolic acidosis and become oliguric and then anuric. As the cardiac output drops the patient may begin to lose cognitive function and will drift into lower levels of consciousness followed by unconsciousness. It is inappropriate to have patients being treated palliatively on cardiac monitors but were they to be monitored, there are several possible terminal stage ECG changes – such as heart blocks and ventricular arrhythmias – before the patient becomes asystolic and dies. These possibilities are important if the patient has an active pacemaker or internal defibrillator as these may be triggered by terminal arrhythmias, hence they need to be deactivated once the patient is in the palliative phase.

SYMPTOMS

Patients at the end of their lives are often troubled by intractable symptoms. Poor quality of life in the terminal stage is the result of uncontrolled symptoms (Stewart 1989). Much can be done to relieve the symptoms and when deliberating symptom relief it is important to consider the causes of the symptoms. It can be seen in Box 12.4 how the symptoms are broadly a consequence of low cardiac output and resultant attempts by the heart to compensate.

Box 12.4 End Stage Heart Failure Symptoms and their Causes

Symptoms	Cause
Breathlessness	Low cardiac output. Raised left atrial pressure and compensatory pressure changes in lungs. Not usually hypoxia but can be if 1) interstitial fluid retention in lungs or 2) anaemia. Possible metabolic acidosis.

Box 12.4 (Continued)

Orthopnea, paroxysmal nocturnal dyspnoea and cough	Right heart unable to cope with increased venous return/pressure when flat.
Fatigue	Low cardiac output. Poor muscle blood perfusion. Poor storage and utilisation of blood in muscles. Also anaemia.
Peripheral oedema	Low cardiac output. Compensatory hormonal activation. Water and salt retention. Poor circulation and venous return.
Pain, itching and agitation	Possible tissue hypoxia. Effects of other symptoms (immobility, constipation, etc.).
Dizziness	Low cardiac output and arterial hypotension. Possible drug-induced orthostatic hypotension.
Palpitations	Possible arrhythmias or reflex sinus tachycardia. Possibly anxiety. Increased ectopy, possibly due to electrolyte balance or structural changes.
Nausea, loss of appetite and cachexia	Low cardiac output. Reduced blood flow to GI tract. Poor absorption from gut. Also poor absorption and metabolism of medication.
Anxiety, depression, confusion, memory loss and insomnia	Poor cardiac output. Brain hypoperfusion. Cortisol changes. Psychological and social influences. Tissue hypoxia. Impaired drug metabolism.

CONTROLLING SYMPTOMS

The common physiological theme that links end of life symptoms is that they are either a direct or indirect response to the progressively worse cardiac output. This situation is not going to be solved and so the underlying cause of the symptoms will not be removed. Additionally, the psychological effects of being in the process of dying are not going to be solved for the patient. The best that can be hoped for is that the symptoms are palliated – they are managed and reduced to as low a level as possible for that patient.

Box 12.5 Symptom-relieving Interventions

Breathlessness	diuretics, nitrates, opioids, oxygen, saline nebulisers, CPAP, NIPPV, fan, breathing exercises, adaptation and coping strategies
Insomnia and anxiety	sedatives, sleep aids
Pain	opioids
Nausea	anti-emetics, diet modification
Constipation	laxatives, diet modification
Weight loss	liquid food supplements

BREATHLESSNESS

Patients with heart failure have usually had chronic exertional breathlessness for some time but in the end stage of heart failure, as their cardiac output drops, their breathlessness is present even at rest. The patient may also have orthopnoea, paroxysmal nocturnal breathlessness and haemoptysis as part of this increased breathlessness. The causes of breathlessness are multifactorial and complex, as we discussed in Chapter 6, and alleviating the symptom can be complex.

The first consideration is whether the patient is hypoxic. Usually, in heart failure patients are not hypoxic but they may be hypoxic when they are acutely unwell or at the end stage. If the patient is hypoxic then the addition of low flow oxygen (24 %) can be therapeutic. However, if the patient is not hypoxic it will not have any benefit beyond possible psychological effects – that may be positive or negative. If the patient is hypoxic then pulmonary oedema should be considered a likely cause, in which case measures to remove fluid and reduce afterload will help, such as higher dose diuretics and nitrates, as well as morphine. These may, however, reduce blood pressure further and this may have deleterious effects, so an individual risk–benefit decision should be made.

Morphine is very effective in reducing chronic severe breathlessness. This is due to several mechanisms: as well as being excellent in reducing afterload it gives the patient a sense of dissociation, which is very beneficial in allowing the patient to relax – with consequent beneficial effects for the overactive adrenaline system. Initially, morphine can be used in oral long-acting preparations (*MST*) with short-acting morphine (*oramorph*) for acute breathlessness. If the patient is not able to take oral medicines then a syringe driver may be required. As always with morphine, an anti-emetic will need to be used in addition and there is a trade between symptom relief and negative effects such as drowsiness and constipation.

Peripheral fluid retention is a sign that preload is high and this will eventually affect breathing by increasing volume and pressure. As well as diuretics, ACE-inhibitors and spironolactone reduce breathlessness by reducing preload. Since they help breathlessness it is logical that stopping these drugs could lead to a worsening of this symptom and for this reason they should be continued even during the palliative stage, if at all possible.

Raised preload as a result of increased venous return is linked to orthopnoea and paroxysmal nocturnal dyspnoea. As well as the drugs noted above, the patient may need help with physical adaptations. For example, a bed with a head that can be raised is very helpful and can usually be supplied through the NHS in palliative care. Nocturnal symptoms can sometimes be overcome by using a sleeping tablet or adding a nitrate, such as buccal suscard, before bed. Paroxysmal nocturnal dyspnoea, cough and haemoptysis are a result of abnormally high lung pressure and the production of metabolic by-products. Supportive measures such as drugs to reduce lung secretions, for example hyoscine, can be of some use, as can physical manoeuvres as directed by a physiotherapist. Bronchodilators can help some breathless patients but there is a need to be wary of tachycardia regarding higher doses of salbutamol as this will decrease diastolic filling time and lead to the worsening of symptoms. If a chronic cough develops, then normal saline nebulisers can help expectoration and cough suppressants, such as codeine linctus or oramorph, can be helpful.

GASTROINTESTINAL SYMPTOMS

As the cardiac output fails the gastrointestinal tract is undersupplied with blood. Chronic over-activation of the adrenaline system, in an effort to increase cardiac output, means the gastrointestinal system receives a disproportionally lower amount of this lowered cardiac output – as blood is supplied differentially to the heart and brain – resulting in several symptoms.

In end-stage heart failure the loss of muscle bulk and weight loss is often marked as the metabolism slows, appetite declines and food absorption falls. Cachexia is associated with a very poor prognosis (Akashi et al. 2005). As we have seen, loss of muscle worsens breathlessness as does anaemia, so this situation is to be avoided or palliated. It is helpful to get the advice of a dietitian. Practical assistance may be needed – such as smaller meals, more frequent meals and change of food types or texture. There may be some value in using liquid-based supplements and fat soluble vitamins. Cholesterol levels are likely to drop and cholesterol lowering agents may require suspension. The use of artificial feeding is generally not a good idea as it fails to recognise that the patient is dying. It is not acceptable to avoid fluids, however, if the patient is unable to assist themselves.

Nausea and vomiting is not as universal a problem in heart failure palliative care compared with cancer palliative care. Nausea is a frequent symptom but vomiting less so. None the less it is still a frequent symptom. The mechanisms are a combination of reduced blood supply to the bowel, changes to nerve activity in the bowel and the effects of medications and psychological distress to do with symptoms and dying.

It is wise to consider which medications are no longer vital and remove those that are not to reduce the chance of causing nausea. It is not advisable to withdraw medication that may be maintaining blood supply to the bowels, such as ACE-inhibitors, unless there are other reasons for doing so.

Anti-emetic medications can have a role to play in heart failure although they are unlikely to do more than ease the symptoms to a degree, as they are unable to address the underlying cause. Drugs such as metoclopramide, haloperidol, domperidone and prochlorperazine are fine to use but cyclizine can worsen heart failure and should be avoided. Non-pharmacological interventions such as visiting, counselling and the hospice can all have a positive effect on patients' ability to cope psychologically and therefore also on symptoms such as nausea and vomiting.

PAIN RELIEF

It is unclear the extent to which pain is a common symptom in end-stage heart failure: some studies suggest it is present in as much as 70 % of patients but other studies put the figure much lower. The likelihood of having pain does increase though as the heart fails and other organs start to become ischaemic. The mechanisms of pain are multifactorial and the psychological component should not be underestimated.

In these circumstances, the experience of the palliative care approach to pain relief can be valuable. The World Health Organization's analgesia ladder provides a framework for up-titrating pain relief as required – see Box 12.6. Remember that NSAIDs can worsen heart failure and should be avoided. We have already seen how opioids can be useful for palliation of breathlessness in heart failure and the same graduated response can be used to treat pain. Whenever opioids are used constipation

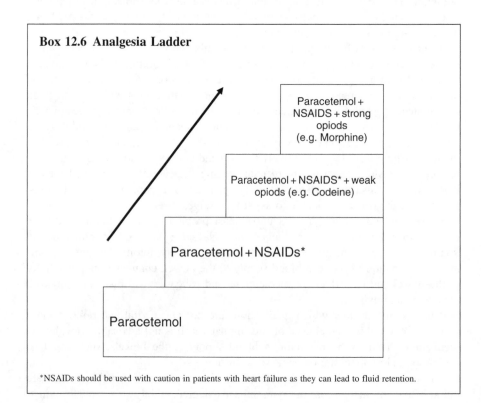

Box 12.6 Analgesia Ladder

Paracetemol + NSAIDS + strong opiods (e.g. Morphine)

Paracetemol + NSAIDS* + weak opiods (e.g. Codeine)

Paracetemol + NSAIDs*

Paracetemol

*NSAIDs should be used with caution in patients with heart failure as they can lead to fluid retention.

should be considered as a highly likely side-effect and nausea as a probable side-effect. The help of other members of a multi-disciplinary team – such as physio-therapists and occupational therapists – can be invaluable in helping to reduce pain.

COGNITIVE IMPAIRMENT AND CONFUSION

As cardiac output drops the brain receives a smaller blood supply and this can lead to symptoms. It is common for patients with advanced heart failure to report a worsening of cognitive functioning and memory and this can deteriorate further during the end stage of their condition. Confusion can also result from this process or can be a result of electrolyte imbalances, drug toxicity or acidosis.

END OF LIFE AND CARDIAC MEDICATION

In palliative care, all medications should be reviewed and non-essential medication should be removed. The physiology of heart failure means that there are particular issues with stopping some of the medications used.

Box 12.7 Stopping Medication in End Stage Heart Failure

Drug type	Examples	Issues
Blood thinning agents	Aspirin, clopidogrel, dipyridamole, Sinthrome, warfarin	Stopping increases the risk of thrombotic events such as heart attacks and strokes.
Cholesterol-lowering drugs	Statins, fibrates	Stopping may increase the risk of thrombotic events.
Anti-anginals	Nitrates, calcium channel blockers, beta-blockers, potassium channel agonists	Stopping may increase the frequency of angina.
Anti-arrhythmic and rate control drugs	Amiodarone, verapamil, sotalol, digoxin	Stopping may increase the risk of arrhythmias
Beta-blockers	Bisoprolol, carvedilol	Stopping may lead to reflex tachycardia and haemodynamic instability.

Box 12.7 (Continued)

Drug type	Examples	Issues
ACE-inhibitors, angiotensin II receptor blockers and aldosterone antagonists	Ramipril, lisinopril, enalapril, perindopril, candesartan, spironolactone, eplerenone	Stopping may lead to over-activity of RAAS system and increased breathlessness and fluid retention.
Diuretics	Furosemide, bumetanide, bendroflumethiazide, metolazone	Stopping may increase breathlessness and fluid retention.

Generally speaking, most clinicians would stop the preventive medications (blood thinning agents, cholesterol-lowering agents and anti-arrhythmics) but continue with the drugs that have a haemodynamic or symptomatic effect (beta-blockers, RAAS active drugs and diuretics). However, it may be necessary to reduce the doses of these drugs to take into account the patient's worsening condition. If drugs such as beta-blockers or ACE-inhibitors are to be stopped they should be reduced first, rather than just stopped, to reduce the chance of a rebound effect.

RESUSCITATION ISSUES

End-stage heart failure is a terminal condition. Once this is recognised it is sensible to think about resuscitation, as patients with heart failure will often end up in an acute healthcare setting where active resuscitation will be the default position if the patient's wishes or circumstances are not known. Patients' wishes vary considerably on this issue. Some patients want to be left alone whereas others want all possible interventions. Even if the patient opts for the latter, it should be explained to them with great sensitivity why this may not be appropriate. For example, no anaesthetist or ICU specialist is going to be in favour of ventilating someone with irreversible, severe heart failure. For patients in their own home resuscitation is less likely to be an issue, with the very important exception of patients with internal defibrillators.

It is common for patients in the final stages of their lives to have arrhythmias such as ventricular ectopy, ventricular fibrillation, fine ventricular fibrillation, or agonal rhythms, before asystole. If the patient has an active internal defibrillator then some of these rhythms will lead to defibrillation. In the context of a patient who is dying, this can be very upsetting. It is also inappropriate as the therapy is no longer required or useful.

In these circumstances, internal defibrillators should be deactivated. This can de done temporarily with a powerful magnet but modern internal defibrillators will reset themselves when the magnet is removed (this feature is to avoid accidentally switching off the machine). To deactivate the device completely it must be done using a programmer, operated by a cardiac technician. There is concern that as the number of implanted internal defibrillators increases the ability to get hold of a technician to do this will become harder.

One cannot assume that patients will want a particular course of action. Nor does this necessarily relate to clinicians' perceptions. The SUPPORT study found that clinicians inaccurately predicted their patients' wishes in 24 % of cases overall; and 50 % of hospitalised, severely ill heart failure patients preferred treatment aimed at quality of life rather than longevity (The SUPPORT Principal Investigators 1995). Patients' wishes can of course change over time and be dependent on circumstances – the same study found changes either way over follow-up – which demonstrates the importance of open communication.

PSYCHOLOGICAL AND SPIRITUAL DIMENSION

Dying is a natural and inevitable process. It is not something most people dwell on but as people get older or have more health problems they give it more thought. People's personalities are all different and their experiences of other people's deaths affect them differently. This means that people approach death in different ways – some are resigned, some accepting, some pessimistic, some hopeful, some angry and some disbelieving. All dying patients should be considered to have particular psychological and spiritual needs.

Does this mean that only experts can support them? No, it means the opposite. Everyone must support them but each person is likely to do so in different ways depending on their experiences, skills and personality.

The clinician, should offer support in the form of professional advice, referrals to others and knowledge of how to get things done, at the same time as providing a non-family person for the patient to express themself to and to share the experience with. The clinician should be able to provide insight and context, having already experienced many deaths, and offer hope as to how the death can be made comfortable and the process supported.

FAMILY AND CARERS

It is important not to forget about the patient's family and carers in palliative care situations. They spend much more time with the patient than any clinician does and their attitudes and approach will be more significant for the patient. They are likely to be as upset as the patient by the dying process. Doing something often becomes their way of coping. They need support along with the patient but their needs will differ. Caregivers of patients with heart failure have a high prevalence of depression, which correlates with the severity of the patient's disease (Hooley et al. 2005).

Family members and carers can be helped in different ways. For some, practical advice in clinical matters and referrals for devices and support are important. For some, the assistance of support groups and bereavement counselling can be helpful. For others this is not the case. Do not feel it is necessary to provide all the answers – regular contact, kindness and interest go a long way.

SPECIALIST PALLIATIVE CARE

Palliative care services were developed by specialists working with patients dying of cancer and have shown how patients can be given dignity and ease at the end of their life. It is widely recognised that the palliative care model should be available to all patients with a terminal condition, regardless of the disease (NICE 2003; Gibbs et al. 2006).

Using a palliative care approach does not, however, mean transferring the patient to specialist palliative care services. Palliative care specialists have an important role to play in helping to set up guidelines, providing expert advice and, sometimes, extra facilities. However, all nurses have a professional code of conduct obligation to provide palliative care as required for their patients. Suddenly aborting heart failure services and transferring patients to palliative care teams is neither sensible nor preferable. Patients will benefit from the support of both and there should be a joint approach based on the patient's individual needs and wishes and that of their family.

In the majority of cases, this will be in the form of support allowing them to die at home. Health service policy is moving quickly towards this model and resources are following. There is much variation with regard to what is available locally for patients in different areas and the palliative care team can offer good advice and contacts to support them.

Occasionally, patients may request hospice care. The benefits of hospice are a safe environment with expert help and the opportunity to take stock. However, this would be an unusual request for heart failure patients, especially if they are inpatients (Fried et al. 1999). Access to these facilities is uneven across the country and in some areas there is a clear inequality favouring cancer patients. The reasons for this are historic as the palliative care movement was begun and remains dominated by people with a particular interest in cancer, while bed numbers are limited and the demand high. It is unlikely that heart failure patients would overrun the existing hospice provision as half of heart failure patients tend to die suddenly, a high number are admitted acutely to hospital and a number will not wish to use the hospices out of choice. There is probably a greater demand for day hospice and hospice-at-home-type services.

An additional complicating factor is that palliative care services have often been dependent on private and charitable funding. They have been under-resourced by the health service and their workers are therefore often envious of the health service resources. None the less, these days the majority of hospices do receive funding through PCTs and a percentage of this funding is dedicated to providing services for non-cancer patients.

The situation is changing, however, and palliative care specialists increasingly recognise that they should provide palliative care more generally and not only cancer care. To achieve this goal, the relevant specialists must move forward, both nationally and locally. In recent years there have been a number of conferences on heart failure and palliative care. New tools such as the End of Life Care Programme, Liverpool Care Pathway and the Goals Standards Framework are making the implementing of a palliative care model for heart failure patients considerably easier.

Box 12.8 Useful End of Life Web Links/Documents

http://www.goldstandardsframework.nhs.uk/
http://eolc.cbcl.co.uk/eolc
http://www.lcp-mariecurie.org.uk/

SERVICE ISSUES

Most areas of the country have established and resourced palliative care services, although what is available locally varies a great deal. These services include specialists in palliative care, Macmillan nurses, hospices, Marie Curie nurses, district nurses and voluntary organisations.

It would make no sense to set up stand-alone services to provide palliation for heart failure patients, given the cost involved and the existing large body of experts with the necessary skills, experience and resources.

This is not to say that the needs of heart failure patients are synonymous with those dying of other conditions. Indeed, they have particular and distinct needs. As each patient's needs are so different as death approaches, care should always be individualised. Patients who are dying probably have more in common with each other than we sometimes realise, especially in the spiritual and psychological dimensions.

What is required are the links, processes and networks that enable patients to access the services they need as and when they need them. This is difficult to organise as it needs to operate on different levels. Individual contact is crucial. Organisational support and mechanisms for formal assessments and review of services make a difference. Government initiatives are changing health service policy by funding service improvement projects around the country, which can be used as examples of best practice when successful.

Box 12.9 Heart Failure/Palliative Care Multi-Disciplinary Team

- patient
- family and carers
- primary care team
- palliative care team
- heart failure team
- Macmillan nurses
- Marie Curie nurses
- voluntary sector

Part IV Policy and Service Issues

13 Policy Framework

This chapter will outline how heart failure has become a health priority. Department of Health policy documents and the scope of professional guidelines will be discussed. Although the emphasis is on the United Kingdom, some comparisons will be made with other countries for illustrative purposes.

HISTORICAL PERSPECTIVE

We have seen how heart failure is not a newly discovered condition but has been known for centuries. It is, however, becoming more of a concern for the health service because the number of patients with heart failure is increasing and the range of treatments available is expanding. In Chapter 2 we discussed how the number of patients with heart failure is increasing due to people living for longer and primary cardiac event survival. In Part III the ways in which treatment has a positive impact on prognoses were explained.

Matching the higher demand for heart failure care has been a greater interest in recent years in redesigning health services to meet this demand and to supply a more clinically-effective and cost-efficient service. Several strands of public policy and professional changes have come together. The high cost of hospital admissions, long stays and re-admission rates of patients with heart failure has led to an interest in better discharge planning and follow-up after discharge. There have been drives to change the nature of follow-up services with the greater involvement of nurses. Variations in care have led to thinking about care pathways, targets and standards. There has been an effort to bring the evidence base more directly into clinical practice.

Over the past ten years the policy frameworks within which heart failure services are delivered have undergone a substantial change. An understanding of these issues is important to appreciate how to maximise the benefits for patients.

NATIONAL SERVICE FRAMEWORKS

The Department of Health began its policy overhaul with the NHS Plan in 2000 (Department of Health 2000a). This document stated the overall strategy for government health policy and the NHS. One of its principal concerns was the lack of national standards and the need to reduce inequalities of care within the NHS. In order to provide standards, the National Service Frameworks for specific priority conditions or patient groups were to be the key planning documents for staff and managers.

The National Service Framework for Coronary Heart Disease was one of the first to be published in 2000 (Department of Health 2000b). Coronary heart disease was chosen as a priority because of the high occurrence of this disease, its impact on mortality and the variations in care across the country. The National Service Frameworks give specific targets and a staged time frame in which they are to be met.

It was recognised that meeting the challenges of the National Service Frameworks was going to be difficult in a number of ways. Firstly, greater resources – staff and facilities – had to be put in place. This meant greater funding for services and an effort to recruit and train more specialist staff. Secondly, the government has been very keen on the reform of the NHS. By reform, the government has meant changes to working practices and care systems, with the goals of greater efficiency, flexibility and more patient-orientated services. In order to support the National Service Framework agenda, drive forward reform and share best practice across health economies, the Cardiac Networks (formerly known as Collaboratives) were set up. These act in a similar way to project managers in industry.

The National Service Framework for Coronary Heart Disease, most people would agree, has been generally successful in improving cardiac care. For example, by setting very challenging thrombolysis targets, linking their achievement to the hospital trusts' performance monitoring and putting in place a rigorous audit system, the achievement of those targets has largely been met across the country.

Critics argue that the problem with a national target-driven approach like the National Service Frameworks is that issues that are untargeted never receive sufficient attention or resources. An example of this would be that the original National Service Framework for Coronary Heart Disease did not contain any standards for the care of people with arrhythmias and the United Kingdom's implantation rates for pacemakers and internal defibrillators have lagged well behind those of the United States and Western Europe as these interventions have not been sufficiently resourced. A chapter on arrhythmias was added to the National Service Framework for Coronary Heart Disease in 2004.

Chapter Six of the National Service Framework for Coronary Heart Disease covers heart failure. This contains only the single standard.

Box 13.1 NSF for CHD Standard Eleven

Doctors should arrange for people with suspected heart failure to be offered appropriate investigation (e.g. electrocardiography, echocardiography) that will confirm or refute the diagnosis. For those in whom heart failure is confirmed, its cause should be identified – the treatments most likely to both relieve symptoms and reduce the risk of death should be offered.

The chapter then goes on to give details of issues with regard to diagnosis, treatment, service design and audit of heart failure in both primary and secondary care. To achieve the standard it is expected that primary care teams and hospitals conduct an annual audit to show that all patients with heart failure have had a full investigation and treatment as appropriate.

Critics of the chapter point out that the recommendations are not as strong or specific as in other chapters and the language means it is possible for healthcare providers to achieve the audit requirements with a relatively low level of actual service. The targets do not link clearly to best practice or recommendations that are given in the chapter between the standard and the milestones.

The chapter does, however, provide a basis for service providers and commissioners to plan and develop services for heart failure. The chapter stresses the importance of having protocols in place for heart failure, multi-disciplinary working, the availability of dedicated specialist heart failure services and means to bridge the interface between primary and secondary care.

Supporting and developing the chapter has been the work of the Cardiac Networks. Heart failure has been a specific work-stream within all Cardiac Networks and there have been conferences to discuss best practice and change. Service Improvement Managers from the Cardiac Networks have often been crucial to improving access and waiting times for investigations such as an echocardiography by redesigning services to reduce blocks in the system. Useful, practical documents have also been published, such as *Developing Services for Heart Failure* (Department of Health 2003).

While the chapter can be criticised for not mandating specific targets it would be fair to say the recommendations it contains about the elements of heart failure service provision need to be taken seriously by commissioners and providers. It is the basis on which the Health Care Commission is carrying out reviews of heart failure services around the country.

Box 13.2 NSF for CHD Web Link

http://www.dh.gov.uk/en/Publicationsandstatistics/Publications/Publications PolicyAndGuidance/DH_4094275

PROFESSIONAL GUIDELINES SPECIFIC TO HEART FAILURE

The National Service Framework provides a framework but does not contain a great deal of detail on the clinical aspects of care, cost effectiveness or evidence base. For these, it is necessary to consult the professional guidelines. These are consensus documents issued by expert committees of various national and international professional associations. In the United Kingdom, the NICE guidelines on chronic heart failure were published in 2003 and the Scottish SIGN guidelines were updated in 2007. The European Society of Cardiology (ESC) heart failure guidelines have been developed for Europe while North America has the American College of Cardiology/American Heart Association (AHA/ACC) guidelines and Canadian Medical Association guidelines. All of these documents can be downloaded at the web addresses in Box 13.3.

Not surprisingly, as they are derived from the same evidence base, there is very little difference among the various guidelines. They all provide a detailed, evidence-based justification for all aspects of caring for patients with heart failure. As well as being useful in this positive sense, they are also helpful in highlighting the areas of care where evidence is weak, controversial or missing.

Box 13.3 Professional Heart Failure Guidelines Web Links

http://guidance.nice.org.uk/CG5
http://www.sign.ac.uk/guidelines/published/index.html
http://www.escardio.org/knowledge/guidelines/Guidelines_list.htm?hit=quick
http://www.americanheart.org/presenter.jhtml?identifier=3004550

NICE GUIDELINES

The National Institute for Clinical Excellence is an independent body funded by the United Kingdom government with the purpose of evaluating and advising on best evidence care for patients in the NHS. It provides policy advice after an assessment of the clinical and cost effectivesness of treatments. It sets up committees of experts and interested parties who use standardised evidence-based procedures to evaluate treatments. The results are published and are almost always taken up by the government as policy. NICE guidance in the United Kingdom therefore provides a template against which care needs to be matched by local services.

In 2003, NICE published their guidelines for the care of patients with chronic heart failure. It is worth noting that the guidelines do not specifically relate to acute heart failure and there is relatively little on acute hospital care in the document.

PRIMARY AND SECONDARY CARE

There have been several policy changes related to primary care and the relationships between the different healthcare sectors in recent years. The three that have had the most recent impact are the movement of services out of secondary care, the new GMS contract for GPs and the introduction of the role of community matrons.

MOVEMENT OF SERVICES

Traditionally the local acute hospital has provided both diagnostic and treatment services for conditions such as heart failure. Whilst some of this care is for inpatient admissions, the majority of the care takes place in the outpatient department. The hospital is where the specialist staff have been based – cardiologists, specialist nurses and cardiac technicians.

It has long been recognised that there are several problems with this model. Firstly, hospital-based services have become congested with patients over the years and their ability to expand their supply to meet an increased demand has been limited by resources – not only staff but also practical issues such as clinic time. As a result, the patient may have had to wait some time for an appointment. Service redesign has allowed some of these problems to be reduced – for example, by ring-fencing patients into a dedicated service or clinic and by increasing the number of nurse-led clinics and technician-led investigations. The second set of issues is concerned with the patient's experience of secondary care services. The patient has to get to the hospital and this can be difficult for many heart failure patients. The typical set-up of secondary care outpatient clinics means that the patient will have a relatively limited consultation time, usually only ten minutes. This can be insufficient to provide all the information and education necessary for a complex condition such as heart failure and patients often feel they have not had sufficient time to express and discuss their concerns.

An alternative model is to move some services that have traditionally been provided in secondary care into primary care. Fundamentally, there is very little done in hospital for chronic heart failure that cannot be done in primary care, such as diagnostics, treatment or follow-up.

There are different ways in which services can be moved from the hospital to primary care. One option is that hospital staff and resources can move in an outreach manner to a community clinic or long-term conditions centre for heart failure sessions. Alternatively, services can be based and staffed permanently in such centres. Community-based specialist heart failure nurses can be appointed. Another option would be for existing resources such as GPs and community nurses to be given further training to operate as practitioners with a specialist interest in heart failure. There are advantages and disadvantages of all these options and different options will work better in certain localities.

GMS CONTRACT

We have seen how the National Service Framework for Coronary Heart Disease has largely been successful in meeting its targets for improving aspects of cardiac services performance in hospital trusts. A major way in which this was achieved was by linking these targets to the trust 'star'-grading scheme. Thrombolysis times, surgical waiting times and those of Rapid Access Chest Pain Clinics all had to meet the National Service Framework targets in order to gain stars. A trust with a poor star rating level had several severe sanctions – potentially, greater central financial scrutiny, the sending in of improvement teams, poor publicity and not being able to apply for Foundation Hospital Status.

Several strands were also likely to lead to changes in GP practices. In particular, the government saw an opportunity during negotiations over the new GP contracts for General Medical Services (GMS) to push forward its reform agenda by linking GP remuneration to the achievement of policy objectives. At the same time, Primary Care Trusts have been given the responsibility of ensuring delivery of the National Service Frameworks in their local areas.

The GMS contract came into force in 2004. It is a form of payment by results in that points are allocated for patients and additional points are available if the GP practice reaches a range of administrative and clinical targets for those patients – this is known as the Quality and Outcomes Framework (QOF). A practice that has good data systems and is carrying out care to the agreed targets will receive a greater income than those practices that do not. This incentive worked a great deal better than initially expected and the income of practices after the introduction of the new contract generally has risen substantially.

There are currently three point indicators that relate directly to heart failure. LVSD1 is simply that the practice should have a register of heart failure patients. As long as the practice has up-to-date IT databases it is simple to draw up a register of patients in this way. LVSD2 is achieved as long as the target percentage is reached of patients with left ventricular systolic dysfunction who have had their diagnosis conformed by an echocardiogram. The practices can exempt patients with a long-standing historic diagnosis from this indicator. LVSD3 is achieved if the target percentage is reached of ACE-inhibitors being prescribed for patients with left ventricular systolic dysfunction. Practices can exempt patients from LVSD3 if they are contra-indicated or intolerant of ACE-inhibitors.

It is apparent that these three indicators are a fairly crude way to judge heart failure care. They do not offer any incentive to diagnose and treat diastolic heart failure, there is no mention of beta-blockers or spironolactone, and nor are the education, support and lifestyle treatments of heart failure covered. Before being too critical, it should be noted that targets are always likely to miss important areas and too many targets lead to confusion and divert attention. There is no reason why the QOF point indicators for heart failure cannot change as practice changes. They are just one of many tools to improve performance.

Since the new General Medical Services (GMS) contract, the QOF data show that the number of heart failure patients with an ACE-inhibitor prescription has increased greatly compared with previous audits. This may be due to the importance of ACE-inhibitors now being more widely understood and because more nurses are available to help manage these patients. However, it would be naïve to think that the galvanising effect of the QOF points has not also played a role in the improvement.

COMMUNITY MATRONS

The third policy trend that has had an impact on heart failure provision in recent years is the introduction of community matrons. In the United States, there has been a long history of generic advanced nursing practitioners working alongside specialist nurses. One of the areas in which nurse-led care has been shown to be effective is the support of patients with long-term and chronic diseases. This type of patient tends to have multiple co-morbidities and will use a disproportionate amount of healthcare resources. By implementing a system of closer, nurse-led care of these patients, the aim is to reduce any unnecessary hospital admissions and the number of emergency contacts, whilst improving patients' quality of life and other outcomes. This relies on nurses to look after complex cases and requires the co-ordinating of services, detecting problems early and implementing care solutions. In the United States, a private company, Evercare, developed a community model of care, which has aroused interest in the Department of Health regarding nurse-led community care for long-term conditions.

In the United Kingdom, the government made a decision to implement a community matron model. There was no widespread piloting of this model and it would be fair to say that it has raised a number of concerns. Some primary care trusts have been meeting the Department of Health directives on community matrons by rebadging existing staff or unilaterally moving staff into these roles. Some areas have recruited large teams and others have very few matrons. The grading has varied among areas. Perhaps the two biggest concerns are that the roles and responsibilities are not yet defined clearly or consistently and that the matrons often feel under-trained.

In the United States, advanced practice is a regulated qualification that requires a Clinical Master's Degree. In the United Kingdom, despite years of debate, neither the UKCC nor the NMC has mandated a definition and requirement for advanced practice registration. It is unclear whether or not community matrons are advanced practitioners. They are certainly being asked to operate at a highly independent clinical level with a great deal of responsibility for care co-ordination and planning. Some areas also expect them to have an advanced clinical role, such as carrying out clinical examinations after a two-day course, when clearly this is not going to provide the competence that a Clinical Master's Degree confers. In some areas, community matrons have to push relentlessly to be sent on any sort of training for their role while they are already in post, seeing to patients.

How does this affect patients and services for heart failure? Clearly, chronic heart failure is a long-term condition and patients with heart failure often have other co-morbidity. They would therefore fit the criteria for community matron involvement, so it is likely that community matrons will be caring for patients with heart failure.

Not surprisingly, community matrons come from a wide range of backgrounds and only a small minority are likely to have current knowledge of and skill in heart failure management. Occasionally, where they work in teams, those with specialist knowledge lead the team in particular clinical areas. Being a generalist is implicit in their role, which can be seen to have some similarities in this regard to the role of GPs. It does mean, however, that they will need specialist assistance in areas such as heart failure. As they have to cover such a wide spectrum of diseases, it would not be reasonable to expect them to know the evidence base and treatments, guidelines and protocols in the same detail that a specialist heart failure nurse would. They will, however, be very useful in keeping in close contact with patients, ensuring that the care provided is as per local heart failure protocol and reducing some of the burden on heart failure specialist nurses' caseloads.

Another point is that community matrons are deliberately given small caseloads, usually a maximum of 30–50 patients. This compares with several hundred for a typical heart failure specialist nurse. The reason for this disparity is that the community matrons' level of contact with their patients is much greater. This originates from a concept known as the Kaiser Pyramid, in which 20 % of patients take up 80 % of the resources in chronic disease. It is perfectly sensible to try and improve the outcomes for those patients by concentrating resources. It does mean, though, that community matrons are not available to care for the bulk of the patients. In heart failure care, this would mean patients with mild and moderate heart failure receiving no community matron involvement as they would focus on patients with severe heart failure. It is important that patients with mild or moderate heart failure do receive good care because they will eventually become the severely ill patients of the future, and providing services early postpones that eventuality.

Once the role of the community matron is established and developed it should provide an opportunity for better care for the more severely affected patients with heart failure. It will provide extra support for existing heart failure services and perhaps free up more time for these services to provide better care for patients who are at an earlier stage in their disease progression. As there is so much local variation, the way in which community matrons and heart failure services work together will require local solutions.

FUTURE DEVELOPMENTS

All of the public policies on heart failure discussed in this chapter have been implemented within the past seven years. It is highly likely that the future will also bring many changes in policy. What is certain is that public policy will continue to be made in the context of clinical advances, financial constraints and public opinion.

The clinical advances most likely to change practice are the increased use of new generations of devices (pacemakers, defibrillators and cardiac assist devices) and, possibly, stem cell therapies. At the same time, there may be a decline in the use of surgery for procedures such as cardiac transplants.

It seems probable that there will continue to be a move towards more community-based, easily accessible and flexible heart failure services. Patients, not surprisingly, are insisting that services are run with their convenience as a priority and not that of the clinicians or managers. Community-based services are proving both popular and clinically effective. It would be hard to imagine that there will not continue to be a role for the hospital in providing care for the acutely ill heart failure patient.

What is less clear is who will be providing these services. Professionally, it is likely to be nurses who will run services in the community, with referral to other professionals and hospital specialists as indicated. What type or level of nurse this will involve is more open to question.

It also isn't certain in which health service framework this will be provided. At present, all United Kingdom political parties are committed to a National Health Service but the nature of the NHS is changing, with some commentators seeing the future role of the NHS more as a commissioner of services or conduit to services, rather than as a provider. This model is already in use with the primary care trust-funded but privately-run Community Treatment Centres. However, no matter what the structure of the NHS, or even if it changes to a health system funded either by social or private insurance rather than taxation, there will always be a need for heart failure services. Heart failure patients will continue to require care and there is no doubt that heart failure services are a lot more cost-effective than doing without them.

14 Service Issues

This chapter considers the different ways that a heart failure service can be delivered, which professionals should be involved, the most efficient and cost-effective way to run the service, and the issues and problems commonly encountered. It will also provide practical advice on the different aspects of running a heart failure service.

HEART FAILURE SERVICES

The need to have local, dedicated heart failure services has been recognised in Chapter 6 of the National Service Framework for Coronary Heart Disease and the NICE guidelines for Chronic Heart Failure. Having such a service is a quality indicator used in the audits of the Health Care Commission and European College of Cardiology Cardiovascular Nursing Council. The reason that dedicated heart failure services are seen as the preferable model is that they are now proven to be effective whereas the traditional systems had well-documented problems.

TRADITIONAL SERVICES

In the United Kingdom, patients with heart failure were often managed solely by their GP. If a patient's symptoms were difficult to manage, they might be referred by their GP to the local cardiology outpatients' clinic for advice. If the patient became acutely unwell they were admitted to the local hospital. This admission would be under the care of the on-call medical consultant, usually a general physician, who may or may not refer the patient to the cardiologist. The patient would be discharged back to their GP once stabilised, sometimes with further outpatient follow-up, sometimes without.

There were several potential flaws in this system. Firstly, the patient might never be seen by a clinician with a special interest in heart failure and so might have missed out on an assessment for further treatment. Secondly, there was a potential gap between primary and secondary care. Thirdly, the system was essentially responsive rather than proactive, dealing with problems once they had arisen rather than trying to prevent them. Fourthly, there was potential for variation in quality of treatment as there were no standards against which to compare a service. Fifthly, there were often delays and blocks in the system due to its complexity. These problems had the combined effect of patients with heart failure often receiving poorly co-ordinated and sub-optimal care for their condition.

There was a consensus that the care of patients with heart failure needed to be improved and this is reflected in Chapter 6 of the National Service Framework for Coronary Heart Disease. This encouraged the setting up of dedicated specialist heart failure services as research showed that patients managed in this way had fewer hospitalisations and better outcomes (Hanumanthu et al. 1997). Although this model has been adopted across most of the country, it is not universal. If specialist heart failure clinics are absent there is still much that can be done to improve services, especially at a practice level. The new GMS contract rewards practices for fully diagnosing, treating and monitoring heart failure patients. Whilst this targeting has many positive aspects, it must be noted that the potential pitfall with this system is that it is likely that smaller and single-handed practices will lag behind larger practices in the provision of dedicated clinics or services, potentially continuing a postcode lottery.

SPECIALIST HEART FAILURE SERVICES

Specialist heart failure services can be provided using different models: community- or hospital-based and physician- or nurse-led. The services may be hospital-based with or without community outreach, or be community-based with or without a hospital in reach. Physician-led services may be offered through a hospital consultant, usually a cardiologist and possibly a heart failure specialist, or through a general practitioner with a specialist interest (GPwSI). Nurse-led services are usually run by a heart failure specialist nurse, who will often also be an advanced practitioner. There is no reason why services could not be run by suitable allied health professionals. To provide care, services can use hospital clinics, community clinics, telephone follow-up or home visits. Services can be for a limited period following acute admission, or patients can be case-managed over a longer period.

The type of model used will vary to fit the local service needs and existing resources. Some service is better than none and once services are established they tend to find ways to access further resources as needed. A recent survey showed that in the United Kingdom, 75 % of centres offered heart failure management either in hospital, at home or in combination. Although this is better than the European average of 63 %, it still means that a significant proportion of heart failure patients were not receiving a proven successful method of delivering care (Jaarsma et al. 2006). The characteristics of successful programmes are that they are multi-faceted with planned discharges, intensive patient education, support for self-care, medical regime optimisation and ongoing review (Lyratzopoulos et al. 2004; McAlister et al. 2004; Yu et al. 2005).

MULTIDISCIPLINARY TEAM MEMBERS

We have seen how patients with heart failure have different problems and needs. The complexity of the condition means that the expert involvement of a range of professionals can be helpful. Ideally, there would be a formally constituted and dedicated heart failure multi-disciplinary team, which met regularly and managed a caseload co-operatively. In the real world, that model is only likely to be feasible in larger centres. None the less, the principles of multi-disciplinary working can still be used, by ensuring that there are referral routes available to involve other professionals, as necessary. As always, there is no substitute for regular personal contact with other colleagues.

Box 14.1 Multi-Disciplinary Team Members for Heart Failure Services

- physician
- nurse
- physiotherapist
- occupational therapist
- dietitian
- clinical psychologist/counsellor
- exercise physiologist
- cardiac physiologist/technician
- pharmacist
- social worker
- welfare rights advisers

Doctors

There are physicians with a special interest in heart failure – both cardiologists and GPs. Unfortunately, there are not many. Where there is a physician with a special interest in heart failure, they are often ideally placed to be the clinical lead for the service. This is logical because as well as expertise, they are likely to have good contacts and to be in a position of some authority within the organisation.

If no physician with a special interest in heart failure is available then there is a need to have medical supervision from another appropriate source, such as a consultant cardiologist. Bear in mind that many cardiologists have special interests, particularly in percutaneous intervention, so they may not necessarily be that interested or specialise in heart failure. Their level of actual involvement will depend on the type of service offered and the level of skills of the other staff – in particular, whether the nurse has advanced practitioner skills. If they do, then a physician is needed to provide clinical supervision, planning, a second opinion and general oversight. If not, then a physician may be needed more directly.

Nurses

Heart failure services almost always contain nurses and nurses run many services. This is because almost all of the care falls within the domains of nursing. Nurses have proved themselves to be suitable and successful in this role (Jolly 2002). The level at which nurses practise is high and they have a great deal of independence and responsibility (McCormick 1999). Experience of cardiology and of working at a senior and independent level is of great benefit, especially in a nurse-led service, as it is necessary to provide a high level of leadership, including administrative tasks and business cases, in additional to clinical care.

The actual nursing numbers and their skills mix within a service will depend upon the caseload and case mix. In the United Kingdom, there is much variation in the number of nurses within services. Some services might run with three or four nurses whereas others might have just the one. There are clear advantages to working in a team in terms of extra support, supervision, opportunities to train up junior staff, cross cover for absences and offering a wider service.

Nurse-led heart failure services have been around since the early 1980s (Cintron et al. 1983). They have developed since then and in recent years, with an increased policy focus on heart failure, nurse-led clinics and the expansion of nursing roles have become common to most United Kingdom localities. This has been given impetus by research that has shown that care from specialist heart failure nurses has improved re-admissions, length of stay, mortality and cost effectiveness compared with standard care (Blue et al. 2001; Palmer et al. 2003).

Clinical Psychologists and Counsellors

In Chapter 6 we noted the high rates of anxiety and depression in patients with heart failure. Recognising and treating these issues is important, as outcomes for these patients are worse than for those who are not anxious or depressed. An experienced clinician should readily recognise when a patient is anxious or depressed. A simple screening tool, such as the Hospital Anxiety and Depression (HAD) Score, can help to quantify this impression. Where patients have these conditions the involvement of psychologists can be invaluable. Patients may also require medications, such as anti-anxiety medication and anti-depressants, and in severe cases referral to psychiatric services.

The standard process of educating the patient about their condition and providing coping and adaptation tools, along with giving the patient time to express themselves, can in itself be therapeutic. There are, however, patients for whom specialist psychological help is needed to improve coping, either through counsellors or clinical psychologists.

Provision of these services varies widely and the specialists often have a long waiting list. They can provide very specific and practical advice on how to cope with specific anxiety-related symptoms. They can also be used either as part of an education programme or as a one-to-one referral service.

If the heart failure clinician believes that specialist psychological referral is needed it is important to explain this to the patient in order to gain their agreement to the referral. If their approval is is not secured the intervention is unlikely to work and it will be a wasted referral. Some patients are embarrassed to be referred or believe you are making a slur about their mental health, which you are not. Others feel it is very nebulous and wouldn't be useful to them. The evidence is that 'talking therapies' are at least as effective as anti-depressants.

Dietitians

Many patients with heart failure can benefit from the expertise of the dietitian. The first group who may benefit is patients who are obese. We have seen how there is an obesity paradox with regard to weight in heart failure. None the less, if patients are obese it is often found that their symptoms, such as breathlessness and fatigue, are much worse. There is, therefore, value in reducing a patient's weight. It could be argued that any clinician can give weight reduction advice and that referral to a dietitian should be reserved for patients with complex or resistant obesity. A counter-argument is that the advice of a dietitian should be built into heart failure programmes for all patients. Access to dietitians will be dependent on local resources.

The other group of patients who will need the help of a dietitian are those with advanced heart failure and who are developing a poor appetite, muscle loss and cardiac cachexia. For these patients, a higher protein diet and advice on protein supplements and size of meals can be an important part of maintaining a reasonable functional status.

Pharmacists

In Chapter 10 we saw how patients with heart failure are likely to have polypharmacy and we also know heart failure patients are more likely to be elderly. This raises certain issues with regard to their medication – that of concordance, interactions and effectiveness. Pharmacists can be very helpful in supporting patients with medications management and devices to aid concordance. Primary care trusts have pharmacy advisers and they will often carry out home visits as well as provide telephone advice. Hospitals all have pharmacists who specialise in different areas.

Physiotherapists

The role of the physiotherapist in heart failure is becoming more important as more is discovered about the role of skeletal muscles in heart failure. As well as delivering exercise programmes, physiotherapists are important in helping patients to maintain their functional status. Heart failure patients may have other problems that can be helped by physiotherapy, such as improvements in chronic respiratory breathlessness through pulmonary rehabilitation.

Occupational Therapists

Intractable symptoms are a reality for many patients with heart failure. In these circumstances, adaptation becomes important to ensure a maximisation of what the patient can do. Occupational therapists have the skills to be useful here, not just in a practical sense but also in that patients are often frustrated with their inability to manage tasks. An occupational therapy assessment is usually the first stage in getting patients practical assistance through devices fitted by the social services.

Social Services

There are several circumstances in which patients with heart failure may need help from social services –those who have housing problems, those who have financial difficulties and those in need of personal care packages. Unfortunately, the help that is available from social services sometimes fails to match patients' expectations. It is important to recognise that patients express general frustration with their condition through complaints about services such as social care.

Welfare Rights

As we saw in Chapter 8, the two main financial benefits available to patients are the Disability Living Allowance and the Attendance Allowance (for the over 65s). Unfortunately, patients with heart failure often do not meet the increasingly strict criteria for claiming these benefits. This is because they focus on independent mobility and personal care. Sometimes patients fail to receive the benefits they are entitled to because they are unable to complete the application forms correctly. Welfare rights officers can provide help with filling in the forms so that the patient has the best possible chance of a successful claim.

There are also various specialist independent services to help patients claim benefits. These include the Welfare Rights organisations based in the local authorities and also the Citizens' Advice Bureaux.

FUNDING

The funding of a heart failure service is dependent on the model of the service being set up and the existing resources. In the United Kingdom, services are now commissioned (usually by the primary care trust) from providers (usually the hospital but possibly private companies or the primary care trust itself). This involves an agreement to provide a certain level of funding and to receive a certain service in return for a fixed period.

Costs include capital costs and running costs. Capital costs for heart failure services will usually not be too high. In most cases, existing buildings are used, although there may be running costs associated with them such as leasing or renting and overheads. Similarly, existing equipment is often used or shared. Setting up the service sometimes provides an opportunity to upgrade to new equipment. Essential items include clinical equipment such as sphygmomanometers and stethoscopes, and office equipment such as computers and dictaphones. As part of any budget, maintenance and depreciation costs should be built in. The largest single running cost is staff. The decision about which team members should be dedicated to the service and which should either be commissioned to provide a certain number of hours or referred to, will influence these costs. The typical model is to have nursing staff dedicated to the service and to use the other team members on an *ad hoc* basis by referral.

Staffing levels should reflect the type of service and the size of the caseload. There is no simple formula for this and practice varies considerably. Many areas operate with one specialist nurse to cover a hospital- or PCT-sized area. This is probably not enough. It means that the caseload will have to be managed to allow patients to be discharged. Some other areas operate with a team of nurses. This has the advantage of allowing cross-cover, absence cover, team-working and staff development. It also has the disadvantage of being more costly.

KEY PARTNERS

As well as the NHS, there are other organisations that the service should link with. These might be other public services, such as local government bodies, or charity, voluntary and private-sector organisations. Examples might include patient forums, gyms and patient transport organisations. These are usually set up on a local basis and coverage will be local and will vary from one area to another.

PATIENT PARTICIPATION

Managers and clinicians have traditionally set up health services in a paternalistic manner – that is, telling patients what they need, based on public health data and central policy objectives. Increasingly, it is recognised that there can be a mismatch between what is offered or delivered and what the patients expect or require (Lloyd-Williams et al. 2005). This may be regarding the type of service, the intensity of follow-up, the type of personnel involved or when the service is accessible.

In order to find out what patients want, it is essential to ask them. There are various ways to consult, such as via surveys, focus groups and patients' representatives. Whichever are used, there is an expectation now that the patient's voice is embedded in service design, audit and evaluation. Involving patients does involve some changes in working practices and if it means redeveloping services, there can be costs involved.

There are practical benefits to increasing patient participation for clinicians. It avoids mistakes, reduces complaints and targets resources most effectively. It helps to keep patients happy, to the benefit of everyone.

IDENTIFYING PATIENTS

If a service is being set up from scratch, then how are patients with heart failure to be identified? This will involve some research. Find out the population of the area, whether this is a hospital, PCT or another setting. From this it is easy to use the epidemiological prevalence and incidence data discussed in Chapter 3 to give an idea of the potential heart failure population in the area. This will allow services to be planned.

Next, potential patients can be identified in one of two ways: from hospital or community data. As patients come through the hospital, each episode is recorded and these clinical coding data give a list of those with a diagnosis of heart failure. Also, the records of the cardiorespiratory department at the hospital will give details of echocardiograms that show heart failure. The hospital coronary care unit will have a register of the patients admitted and this can also be checked for patients with heart failure. In the community, heart failure patients can be found through primary care records. As part of the Quality Outcomes Framework, each practice should have a register of patients with left ventricular systolic dysfunction. It is also possible to run searches within individual practices' computer systems to cross reference medications – looking, for example, for patients who have been prescribed beta-blockers, ACE-inhibitors and diuretics. This will give an idea of heart failure patient numbers, although it is a relatively crude way to collect this information and there will be some inaccuracies.

Once established, the easiest way for a new service to find patients with heart failure is simply for them to be referred by other clinicians. The wider the number of clinicians who know about the service and can refer to it, the more patients will be identified.

REFERRALS

There are several issues to consider with regard to referrals: who can make referrals, what the criteria are and what method is used. The choices made will be reflected in the scope of referrals received by the service.

At one extreme, services sometimes only take consultant referrals while at the other extreme, some services will take any referrals, including self-referral. It is possible to limit referrals to consultant level. This should have the advantage of ensuring the patient has been diagnosed correctly, has had the appropriate investigations and has a clear plan of care. It will, however, limit the number of referrals, limit community access and the referrals will tend to be reactive – being made after acute events. Taking referrals from anyone is simple to administer but there are practical difficulties, such as the quality of the referral varying widely (in terms of information received) and there may be more referrals of patients who do not actually have a heart failure diagnosis. People are often worried about 'inappropriate referrals'. To counter this they often set the bar for referrals very high. Doing so will cut down on all referrals, not only inappropriate ones. A middle path between these extremes is to take referrals from all clinicians, once the patient has a confirmed diagnosis. The other determining factor regarding who can refer depends on what type of service you are running – for instance, a community-based service must accept GP referrals.

Clinicians need to know how they should refer patients to the service. There are various methods available – by paper, email, letter or telephone call. A key decision is whether a set form is to be used for referrals. This has the advantage of ensuring certain data are available to the service and reduces inappropriate referrals. It also makes an audit easy. However, insisting on written referrals, especially if it must be on some six-page-long form, will reduce referrals, as many people have neither the time nor inclination to do this. Some referral forms look more like audit tools to make life easier for the service managers. It is preferable to insist only on absolutely essential information – such as the patient's name, NHS number and contact details – as you should always be able to access the notes to check their medical details.

Once the referral system is in place, it is necessary to spread the word about the existence of the service. In hospital, secretaries and ward clerks need to be sent copies of any referral forms to be used, as do the ward sisters and consultants. Don't forget to send copies for the outpatient clinics. Each GP and practice in the locality, health centres and community clinics will need copies. Send a mail shot and if a web-based or computerised intranet is in place, get a copy of the referral form onto that system. It may also be possible to receive referrals electronically. The more personal contacts that can be made with other clinicians, the better. It is human nature that people are more likely to engage with people they have met. There are usually local forums – e.g. practice nurses, district nurses, GPs' protected teaching sessions, hospital audit meetings – that can be attended to meet other clinicians.

Finally, once the service is running it is important to monitor referral patterns. Usually, some clinicians will refer many patients and some, none at all. This is often a legitimate expression of their caseload but sometimes it highlights a problem with knowledge or communication with the heart failure service.

CASELOAD MANAGEMENT

As the referrals start to come in and patients are seen, a caseload is built up. This needs managing to ensure efficiency. How it is managed depends on what service is being run. It can be helpful to categorise the patients into those who are unstable, those who are stable but need optimisation of their treatment and, finally, those who are stable and on full-tolerated treatment. The traditional management of this tripartite division of patients would roughly be inpatient, outpatient and GP; many hospital-based services still run to this model. This allows them to discharge the third category of patients to the GP for follow-up monitoring. The alternative is not to discharge patients but to manage them all within one service, adjusting the frequency of their follow-up accordingly. This allows for population management and a better ability to contact and offer stable patients new treatments and technologies as they become available.

METHOD OF FOLLOW-UP

There is no doubt that by following up patients with heart failure, further admissions can be reduced. The question arises as to what is the best method for this – how often, by what means and by whom? Studies have looked at different models, such as follow-up by telephone, follow-up appointments in hospital outpatient clinics or by home visits, or a combination of these. The reviews might be carried out by specialist nurses or doctors, or by primary care nurses or doctors.

Telephone contact allows a large number of patients to be followed up frequently and easily, at relatively low cost. The disadvantage is that it relies on accurate self-reporting by patients as there is no face-to-face contact at that point. Some patients are not good at this either because they find it hard to judge their symptoms or because their personality means they might either over- or underestimate their symptoms. It makes it more difficult for the person at the end of the telephone to use their clinical judgement as several of the key clinical assessment modalities (sight, smell and body language) are missing.

The evidence base for the value of the telephone follow-up in heart failure is mixed. Self-administered education programmes and follow-up nurse telephone calls in one study had a limited benefit for outcomes (Martensson et al. 2005). Another study of the telephone follow-up (with an ECG facility) found a significant reduction in heart failure re-admissions (Scalvini et al. 2004). The DIAL trial has had the largest number of enrolled patients and used frequent nurse telephone contact (as well as at least three monthly clinic follow-up in both groups). Mortality was similar in both groups but the intervention group had a better quality of life and less frequent hospital admissions (GESICA Investigators 2005). DIAL took stable patients on optimal medical treatment with a large number of social and clinical exclusions. This means that generalising to other heart failure caseloads may be limited. The telephone follow-up may work well for this group but patients with more complex cases may be better off with face-to-face contact.

Clinic visits are the traditional method of follow-up. The problem with them is that getting to the clinic can be difficult for patients and hospital parking almost always is a problem. Clinic appointments may be lost or cancelled and patients may drop off systems. In the traditional medical clinic follow-up appointment, the amount of time allocated is usually ten minutes and the patient will be seen by a junior doctor. For the matter of heart failure, ten minutes is often not sufficient to cover the whole review. Frequently, what is left out is the lifestyle and psychological aspects of the review, which are often rated by patients as the most important.

Outpatient clinics ring-fenced for heart failure patients appear to be better accepted and have better results. It is unclear whether this is because more time is allocated for the patients, the practitioners have a specialist focus, or that the patient feels more valued and validated. Patients report all of these benefits in surveys, along with consistently preferring to see the same regular practitioners. Nurse-led heart failure clinics meet these criteria and are cost effective as they reduce re-admissions, complications and bed days at a relatively low cost (Palmer et al. 2003).

In nurse-led clinics, it is probably sensible to allocate half an hour for follow-up appointments and an hour for first appointments. Follow-up appointments through clinics may not need to be at a hospital as diagnostic testing will already have been carried out. Clinics can be taken into different communities via a number of options, such as basing them at community hospitals, health centres, GP practices or nursing homes. Studies looking at nurse-led heart failure clinics at community hospitals have proved them to be effective in improving drug use and reducing rehospitalisation (Anderson et al. 2005). The practicality of this will, however, depend on local resources and the number of patients involved.

Home visits are usually greatly appreciated by patients. Compared with clinics, they are clearly far more convenient for the patient but a lot less convenient for the clinicians. For the latter, home visits have the advantage of being able to place the patient in their everyday environment, in terms of housing, food, facilities, family and carer support. The main difficulty for the clinician making home visits is that they are time-consuming, especially in rural areas, and that they have to carry any equipment needed. About an hour will need to be allocated for a home visit, on average, with travel taken into account. On a practical level, home visits also carry a small degree of risk if the clinician is unaccompanied. Many organisations offer various services for lone workers such as telephone log-in devices. Another potential problem with home visits is that certain investigations may not be readily available in the community. This is unlikely to be a major issue but there is no doubt that if you work in a clinic based next door to a cardiorespiratory department, it should be quick and easy to secure an ECG or echocardiogram.

Home visits have been shown to be clinically effective. A study of a home-based programme of surveillance and intervention in an elderly heart failure cohort showed reduced hospitalisations and improved functional status (Kornowski et al. 1995). Another home-based study showed reduced re-admissions and out-of-hospital deaths over six months and longer (Stewart et al. 1998, 1999). A combination of nurse-led heart failure clinics plus home-based interventions has been shown in a small, randomised, controlled trial to be twice as effective as the typical care (Thompson et al. 2005). A systematic review of different types of multi-disciplinary interventions in heart failure found that interventions that reduced mortality and re-admission were most effective when delivered, at least in part, in the patient's home (Holland et al. 2005).

Perhaps the ideal situation is to have the freedom and facilities to offer any type of follow-up the patient requires. More practically, all types of follow-up are effective to some degree, so offering whatever service is possible with the resources available is better than nothing. Targeting the higher intensity home visits to those with more severe or complex heart failure, or to those who struggle to attend clinics for mobility or social reasons, is a sensible compromise.

FREQUENCY OF FOLLOW-UP

How often does a patient with heart failure need to be reviewed? This is difficult to answer as it depends on which type of patient is being reviewed. Some patients are clinically unwell or unstable, or they might be struggling to cope psychologically. Others may be asymptomatic and on maximal treatment. Most are located somewhere between those two extremes.

There is no doubt that the transition from hospital to home requires careful management. This is often the time of re-admission. By maximising education and existing discharge programmes, improvements can be made in the patient's quality of life and reductions in emergency department visits (Harrison et al. 2002; Clark & Nadash 2004). Nurse-led transitional care is effective in patients with heart failure (Williams 2003). Discharge planning in heart failure and swift follow-up reduced re-admissions in a meta-analysis of nurse follow-up (Phillips et al. 2005).

Patients who are unwell may need to have contact every day or several times a week. The best predictor of the frequency of follow-up required to maintain stability is renal function (Shah et al. 2005). This also applies to patients who are terminally unwell. These contacts can be time consuming because the issues are unlikely to be simple to resolve and other professionals will need to be liaised with. However, these patients are unlikely to be a large part of the caseload because, on the whole, they will either improve or die relatively quickly. Fluctuations in the number of these patients can affect workload dramatically – it can be very demanding if several patients are at the end-stage of heart failure simultaneously. It is sensible to try to leave some spare capacity in work schedules to cope with any fluctuations. It is also a good idea to audit regularly to see if the case mix is changing over time, and whether there are more or less of these higher-dependency patients. If there is such a change it can be taken as the starting point for a discussion with managers and commissioners about extra resources.

Patients with psychological distress can use a lot of resources and demand regular follow-up, regardless of their physical state. This may seem frustrating but remember that without the heart failure service, they may well be using up their GP's time or even ringing for ambulances and requesting acute admissions. The key is to be realistic about what you can do for them, and listening and providing reassurance where appropriate, after which expert help may be needed from psychologists or mental health teams.

Many services would discharge back to their GP patients who are stable on maximal treatment. This depends on whether the service has a remit to population-manage, in which case the patients can remain on the caseload for review, which could perhaps be carried out once every six months. If patients are being discharged back to their GP, it is worth remembering that their heart failure has not disappeared and they may well be referred back to the heart failure service in the future.

When patients are being supervised during medication optimisation, they will need frequent follow-up. A minimum gap of two to four weeks is needed. If the up-titration process involves the GP adjusting the prescription for each change, then it may be more practical to leave follow-up intervals of six to eight weeks. Bear in mind that frequent clinic visits may be inconvenient for the patient, especially if they are working and if parking at the hospital is difficult or expensive.

For general reviews, a balance needs to be struck between too often and too infrequent. Too frequent contact runs the risk of making the patient feel dependent psychologically and this will also reduce the number of patients that can be seen. Too infrequent contact runs the risk of losing touch with the patient, missing changes in their condition and not having an influence on lifestyle and concordance.

There have been some small studies looking at different ways of delivering care to patients with chronic heart failure. The common finding is that frequent follow-up by a clinician with experience in heart failure results in an improvement in the patients' quality of life and a reduction in emergency admissions. It is unclear what the key variables are in these services but it seems likely that having regular contact with a heart failure expert is reassuring for the patient and provides an opportunity to improve care.

DOCUMENTATION

The old adage that 'care not written is care not given' remains a truism. Clear documentation provides a safety mechanism for patients, staff and managers. They are essential to good clinical governance. It is necessary, when setting up or running a service, to think about what documentation is needed.

The first principles are that documents should be simple to use, have clear purposes and aid, rather than hinder, the smooth running of the service. On a daily basis there is a need to record where staff are (in a diary), when patients are to be seen (in an appointments record), what happens when staff contact patients (on an assessment form) and the outcomes (letters, referrals etc.). As a support to the service, there is also a need for referral guidelines, operating standards and clinical guidelines.

Diaries are usually more efficient if they are electronic rather than paper, in that it is easier for staff to access and co-ordinate them. Using an e-mail-based system has several advantages when planning appointments and meetings. Paper copies can still be printed and stored for record-keeping purposes.

Keeping track of patients' appointments can be challenging, especially if patients are being seen in different locations. Most hospitals computerise this information and primary care settings are also starting to do so via the NHS computer system. It is probably a wise precaution to make a note of patients' appointments on paper about a week beforehand, using a computer printout or by noting appointments in a personal diary.

Some services prefer to use a standardised form for writing clinical notes, while others use hospital notepaper. The important issue is the quality of the notes rather than what paper they are recorded on. Remember to set up a system to record clinical telephone calls and e-mails as well as written communication.

Rather than reinventing the wheel when it comes to documentation, it would be useful to obtain copies from existing services. It is also worth while to examine how they work in practice. While it is tempting to use the most extensive and thorough documents – some care pathways seem to be the length of a dissertation – if half of the pages are never filled in, this shows that the practitioners actually find those pages of no help or importance.

Documents are rarely generated in isolation. They will need to fit the corporate style of the organisation and there may be procedures in place that require the use of existing documents or form templates. Larger organisations have committees that oversee the style and content of documents, especially those that are for public information. It is important to check local requirements.

All heart failure services will need to hold some of their own records. If patients are able to phone the service directly there will not be time to retrieve their hospital notes – and some information needs to be at hand. Needless to say, this must be held securely and in keeping with local record-keeping and data protection policies.

For any service based in hospital, or providing in-reach to a hospital, dealing with hospital notes is often problematic. Notes can be incomplete, missing, filed incorrectly or simply not turn up on time when requested. The value of a good relationship with medical secretaries and the medical records department cannot be overstated.

Ideally, there would be only one patient record and this would be centralised. When electronic clinical patient records become operational, this will be possible. Until that time, it is necessary to ensure that everyone is informed about shared patients through copying letters and assessments to the hospital records, GP records and any other clinicians involved.

Box 14.2 Essential Documents

- service operating standards
- local heart failure clinical guidelines/protocol/care pathways
- referral form (to the service)
- patient database
- patient records
- telephone records
- diary
- referral forms (to other services)

SERVICE EFFECTIVENESS

All services have to be effective if commissioners are going to continue to support them. Patients have a right to expect effective services and clinicians will naturally want to provide them. Effectiveness is a double-edged concept including both clinical effectiveness and cost effectiveness.

Heart failure services have the advantage of being able to point to an existing body of research that shows how these services have been effective in other locations. These can provide benchmarks and targets against which to judge the effectiveness of local services.

It is important to find out what targets or goals are being set for the service. These should be negotiated with all parties involved in order to be relevant and realistic, and matched to service resources and capabilities. Unfortunately, targets are sometimes imposed from above. Targets are often stated in documents such as local development plans (LDPs) within primary care trusts. Targets are sometimes implicit in other policy documents. Any heart failure service would be very foolish not to pay close attention to Chapter 6 of the National Service Framework for Coronary Heart Disease, the NICE guidelines on heart failure and the reports on heart failure of the Health Care Commission, and tailor their services to match these expectations.

Commissioners and managers are particularly interested in whether services meet targets. To achieve these goals, the service must often be designed or adapted to meet them. For example, if a target is to reduce re-admissions, then research shows that many re-admissions occur shortly after discharge. In order to meet this goal, it is logical that involvement in discharge planning and early follow-up is required. In contrast, if there was a target to reduce the number of new admissions with heart failure, then early diagnosis and treatment through screening of at-risk populations would be needed. You can see how one goal is a reactive, secondary care-led target and the other is a proactive, primary care-led target.

It is important to demonstrate that the goal has been met. This requires audit skills and data collection. This can be time consuming but remember that many data are collected electronically through hospital coding and through the practices' computer systems. Collect audit data regularly and have them ready in prepared graphs that can be adapted and used in presentations to managers and commissioners.

As well as showing with statistics that a service is clinically effective, it is important to place the service in the context of the patient. Is the service meeting the needs of patients and do they value it? The most practical way to obtain this information is through a patient satisfaction survey. Smaller focus groups or patient forums are also an option. This is invaluable in spotting glitches in the system. It is only in recent years that any consistent effort has been made to listen to the patient's voice about services but it is now expected that this will take place when services are assessed by organisations such as the Health Care Commission.

Clinical effectiveness is often considered more straightforward to demonstrate than cost effectiveness, while the latter is often overlooked during presentations on a service. Whilst this is understandable, an effort should be made to consider cost effectiveness because it is one of the more powerful arguments in support of heart failure services.

Ultimately, all healthcare costs money and, therefore, is not cost effective. The cheapest healthcare system is one that sees no patients. However, moving beyond that logical extreme, cost effectiveness can be judged in terms of changes to mortality, morbidity, economic usefulness (returning to work) and quality of life improvements. It can also be considered in terms of more appropriate use of resources.

The costs associated with heart failure have been estimated in numerous analyses. All show that heart failure is a major healthcare cost and likely to rise. The bulk of the costs is incurred in acute hospital admissions. The average length of stay is 10 days. In an economic analysis it was calculated that if a nurse-led heart failure service post discharge reduced heart failure hospital admissions by 50 % then the annual saving in the United Kingdom would be £169 000 for every 1000 patients treated (Stewart et al. 2002). Research has shown that nurse-led heart failure services can reduce inpatient admissions by 30–50 % (Stewart & Horowitz 2003). Reductions in heart failure hospital admissions would also free up hospital bed days for other purposes and reduce bed blocking within the hospital system.

The cost of heart failure in primary care is linked to frequent attendance at the GP practice for symptom review and medication costs. While the medication costs are unlikely to change it may be possible to reduce the number of GP attendances by ensuring greater access to heart failure services. This is a more cost-effective solution and frees up GP time for other purposes.

The cost of setting up and running a heart failure service must be placed against these cost savings. Even if a service was being set up from scratch, it would quickly become cost effective if it took on a typical caseload and achieved the typical improvements in clinical effectiveness.

A meta analysis of research suggests that specialist heart failure services are generally cost effective as well as clinically effective (Ahmed 2002). Modelling based on clinical trials and the usual care results shows that the improvement in drug concordance at specialist heart failure clinics can lead potentially to a fourfold decrease in re-hospitalisations and a halving of mortality (Lyratzopoulos et al. 2004). Early intervention reduces the risk of hospitalisation. It is estimated that 54 % of re-admissions for heart failure are preventable (Michalson et al. 1998). The key factors in this are discharge planning, follow-up arrangements and medication compliance – in fact, up to 64 % of re-admissions may be due to non-compliance (Ghani et al. 1988). Heart failure services improve care for patients with heart failure and are less expensive than standard care.

Box 14.3 Useful Audit Data to Demonstrate Effectiveness of Service

Hospital

- admissions
- re-admissions
- bed days

Service workload

- caseload
- referrals
- referrals by source
- patient contacts
- contact by type
- outcomes
- hospital admissions from caseload
- deaths

Patient demographics

- age
- gender
- race
- heart failure aetiology
- NYHA class
- left ventricular ejection fraction

Medications

- eligible patients on different drugs
- eligible patients on maximum tolerated dose

Heart Failure Clinical Trials Index

Acronym	Title	Date of publication	References in text
AIRE	*Acute Infarction Ramipril Efficacy*	1997	p. 147
ATLAS	*Assessment of Treatment with Lisinopril AND Survival*	1999	p. 147
ANZ-Carvedilol	*Australia – New Zealand Heart Failure Research Collaborative Group Carvedilol Trial*	1997	p. 154
AVID	*Anti-arrhythmic Versus Implantable Defibrillator Trial*	2001	p. 176
BEST	*Beta-Blocker Evaluation Survival Trial*	2001	p. 154
CARE-HF	*Cardiac Resynchronisation Heart Failure Study*	2005	p. 173
CASCADE	*Cardiac Arrest in Seattle: Conventional versus Amiodarone Drug Evaluation*	1993	
CASH	*Cardiac Arrest Study Hamburg*	2000	p. 176
CHARM	*Candesartan in Heart Failure Assessment of Reduction in Mortality and Morbidity*	2003	pp. 150–1
CHARMES	*CHARM-Preserved Echocardiographic Sub Study*	2007	pp. 12, 37
CIBIS-II	*Cardiac Insufficiency Bisoprolol Trial*	1998	p. 153
CIDS	*Canadian Implantable Defibrillator Study*	1993	p. 176
COMET	*Carvedilol Or Metoprolol European Trial*	2003	pp. 153–4
COMPANION	*Comparison of Medical Therapy, Resynchronisation and Defibrillation Therapies in Heart Failure Trial*	2004	p. 173
CONSENSUS-1	*Co-operative North Scandinavian Enalapril Survival Study*	1987	pp. 38–9, 146
COPERNICUS	*Carvedilol Prospective Randomised Cumulative Survival Trial*	2001	pp. 153–4

Continued

Acronym	Title	Date of publication	References in text
DIAL	*Randomised trial of telephone intervention in heart failure by the GESICA Investigators*	2005	p. 217
DIAMOND	*Danish Investigators of Arrhythmia and Mortality On Dofetilide*	1998	
DINAMIT	*Defibrillator In Acute Myocardial Infarction Trial*	2004	
ELITE-1	*Evaluation of Losartan in the Elderly*	1997	p. 151
ELITE-2	*Losartan Heart Failure Survival Study*	2000	p. 151
EPHESUS	*Eplerenone Post-AMI Heart Failure Efficacy and Survival Study*	2003	p. 158
GESICA	*Randomised Trial of Low-Dose Amiodarone in Severe Congestive Heart failure*	1994	p. 163
MADIT	*Multicentre Automatic Defibrillator Implantation Trial*	1996	p. 176
MADIT-2	*Multicentre Automatic Defibrillator Implantation Trial II*	2002	
MDC	*Metoprolol in Dilated Cardiomyopathy*	1993	p. 154
MERIT-HF	*Metoprolol CR/XL Randomised Intervention Trial in Congestive Heart Failure*	1998	p. 153
MUSTIC	*Multisite Stimulation in Cardiomyopathies Study*	2001	p. 173
MUSTT	*Multicentre Unsustained Tachycardia Trial*	1996	p. 177
OPTIMAAL	*Optimal Therapy in Myocardial Infarction with the Angiotensin II Antagonist Losartan*	2002	
PATH-CHF	*The Pacing Therapies for Congestive Heart Failure (PATH-CHF) Study*	2001	
PEP-CHF	*Perindopril for Elderly People with Chronic Heart Failure*	2006	
RALES	*Randomised Aldoctone Evaluation Study*	1999	pp. 157–8
RESOLVD	*Randomised Evaluation of Strategies for Left Ventricular Dysfunction Pilot Study*	1999	pp. 151, 154
SAVE	*Survival and Ventricular Enlargement*	1992	p. 146
SCD-HeFT	*Sudden Cardiac Death in Heart Failure Trial*	2005	p. 177

Glossary and Abbreviations

Afterload	*The pressure against which the left ventricle has to contract*
Akinetic	*Literally, 'not moving'*
Ascites	*Free fluid in the abdomen*
Amyloidosis	*Deposition of amyloid tissue*
Biventricular failure	*Failure of both ventricles*
Brain natriuretic peptide (BNP)	*A stress hormone produced by the failing heart*
Cardiac index (CI)	*The amount of blood pumped out by the heart in a minute, adjusted for body size*
Cardiac output (CO)	*The amount of blood pumped out by the heart in a minute*
Cardiac resynchronisation therapy (CRT)	*Pacing of both sides of the heart*
Cardiomegaly	*Enlargement of the heart*
Cardiomyopathy	*Disease of the heart muscle*
Cardioselective	*Used to refer to beta-blockers that work mainly on beta-1 receptors in the heart*
Cardiothoracic ratio	*Proportion of the area of the lung fields, at their widest point, occupied by the heart shadow on a chest X-ray*
Cardioversion	*Electrical shock to reset the heart rhythm, as an elective procedure*
Chronotrope	*Agent that affects the speed of the heart rate – could be either positive or negative*
Clubbing	*Enlargement of the finger (or toe) tips and nail beds*
Congestive cardiac failure (CCF)	*Alternative name for biventricular heart failure*
Continuous positive airways pressure (CPAP)	*A mechanical device to deliver oxygen to keep airways open – sometimes used in acute heart failure and sometimes for sleep apnoea*
Contractility	*Ability of the heart muscle to squeeze*
Corneal archus	*White ring around the iris that can indicate high serum cholesterol*
Cor pulmonale	*Right-sided heart failure due to respiratory disease*
Cyanosis	*Bluish tinge to extremities or mucous membranes as a result of poor lung gas exchange*
Decompensation	*Term indicating the heart is failing acutely because compensatory mechanisms are overwhelmed*

Defibrillation	*Electrical shock to reset the heart rhythm, as an emergency procedure*
Diastole	*The part of the cardiac cycle where the heart is at rest (not contracting)*
Dilation	*Enlargement of a heart chamber*
E-A ratio	*Flow pattern across the mitral valve, providing a measure of diastolic dysfunction on echocardiogram*
Echocardiogram	*Ultrasound of the heart*
Electrocardiogram (ECG)	*Graphical recording of the electrical activity of the heart*
Endocarditis	*Inflammation of the inner lining of the heart*
Frank-Starling Law	*Law describing the effect of the stretch of the heart fibres on the force of contraction*
Gamma glutamyl transpeptidase (GGT)	*A liver function test that is often raised in alcoholics*
Haemochromatosis	*Disease causing abnormally high iron levels*
Haemodynamics	*Measures of blood movement and pressures*
Hypertrophy	*Muscle enlargement*
Hypokinetic	*Literally, 'moving only a little'*
Impedance cardiography (ICG)	*Monitor to measure pressures within the thorax, blood volumes and cardiac indices*
Inotrope	*Agent that affects the contractility of the heart – could be positive or negative*
Intraventricular septum (IVS)	*The muscular membrane separating the left and right sides of the heart and containing a lot of electrical conduction pathways*
Ischaemia	*Blood supply–demand mismatch*
Jugular venous pressure (JVP)	*Visualised pressure in jugular vein. Useful as JVP is the same as central venous and right atrial pressure*
Laplace's Law	*Law that describes how increased dilation means more wall tension is needed to achieve ventricular ejection in dilated cardiomyopathy*
Left bundle branch block (LBBB)	*Pattern of intraventricular septal conduction delay seen on ECG*
Left ventricular assist devices (LVAD)	*Implantable mechanical pump to support the failing left ventricle*
Left ventricular ejection fraction (LVEF)	*The percentage of blood present in the ventricles ejected from the left ventricle into the circulation during each heart beat*
Left ventricular failure (LVF)	*Subdivision of heart failure, seen both acutely and chronically, with failure of the left ventricle*
Left ventricular systolic dysfunction (LVSD)	*Subdivision of heart failure based on echocardiogram evidence of abnormal contraction*
Metabolic equivalents (METs)	*A method of measuring the effort required to do types of exercise*
Myocardial infarction	*Death of heart muscle, usually due to acute coronary thrombosis*
Myocardium	*The middle muscular layer of the heart*
Myocarditis	*Inflammation of the heart muscle*

NYHA class	*A functional scheme to grade heart failure based on symptoms*
Percutaneous coronary intervention (PCI)	*Revascularisation of coronary arteries by cardiac catheterisation techniques*
Pericarditis	*Inflammation of the outer layer of the heart*
Preload	*Force stretching the heart before it contracts*
Prevalence	*The proportion of individuals within a population who have a disease*
Pulmonary artery catheter	*Tube inserted through the skin and central veins, back to the right side of the heart and through the pulmonary valve to the pulmonary artery*
Pulmonary hypertension	*Raised blood pressure within the pulmonary artery*
Pulmonary oedema	*Raised interstitial fluid within the lungs*
Remodelling	*Changes in shape of heart chambers as a response to injury*
Right ventricular failure (RVF)	*Subdivision of heart failure when the right ventricle fails*
Stroke index (SI)	*Amount of blood pumped out by the ventricle in one heart beat, adjusted for patient's size*
Stroke volume (SV)	*Amount of blood pumped out by the ventricle in one heart beat*
Systemic vascular resistance (SVR)	*Measure of resistance or arterial constriction, calculated by dividing blood pressure by cardiac output*
Systole	*Period of ventricular contraction during cardiac cycle*
Transoesophageal echocardiogram (TOE)	*Echocardiogram performed using a swallowed probe*
Transthoracic echocardiogram	*Echocardiogram performed using a standard approach with a probe placed against the chest wall*
Xanthelasma	*Yellow skin lesion as a result of high cholesterol*

References

Abramson J L, Williams S A, Krumholz H M and Vaccarino V (2001) Moderate alcohol consumption and risk of heart failure amongst older persons. *Journal of the American Medical Association* **285** (15), pp. 1971–1977.

Ades P A (2001) Cardiac rehabilitation and secondary prevention of coronary heart disease. *The New England Journal of Medicine* **345** (12), pp. 892–902.

Ahmed A (2002) Quality and outcomes of heart failure care in older adults: role of multidisciplinary disease-management programs. *Journal of the American Geriatrics Society* **50** (9), pp. 1590–1593.

Ahmed A (2007) A propensity matched study of New York Heart Association Class and Natural History End Points in heart failure. *American Journal of Cardiology* **99** (4), pp. 549–553.

Ahmed A and Allman R M (2003) Alcohol and congestive heart failure. Letter. *Annals of Internal Medicine* **138** (1), p. 75.

Ahmed A, Sims R V, Allman R M, De Long J F and Aronow W S (2003) Racial variations in cardiology care among hospitalized older heart failure patients. *Heart Disease* **5** (1), pp. 8–14.

Ahmed A, Allman R A, Aronow W S and De Long J F (2004) Diagnosis of heart failure in older adults: predictive value of dyspnoea at rest. *Archives of Gerontology and Geriatrics* **38** (3), pp. 297–307.

Ahmed A, Husain A, Love T E, Gambasi G, Dellitalia L J, Francis G S et al. (2006) Heart failure, chronic diuretic use, and increase in mortality and hospitalization: an observational study using propensity score methods. *European Heart Journal* **27** (12), pp. 1431–1439.

Akashi Y J, Springer J and Anker S D (2005) Cachexia in chronic heart failure: prognostic implications and novel therapeutic approaches. *Current Heart Failure Reports* **2** (4), pp. 198–203.

Ali A, Mehra M R, Malik F S, Lavie C J, Bass D and Milani R V (1999) Effects of aerobic exercise training on indices of ventricular repolarisation in patients with chronic heart failure. *Chest* **116** (1), pp. 83–87.

Allan R, Kass M, Glover C and Haddad H (2007) Cellular transplantation: future therapeutic options. *Current Opinion in Cardiology* **22** (92), pp. 104–110.

Anand I S, MacMurray J J V, Whitmore J et al. (2005) Anaemia and clinical outcome in heart failure. *Cardiology Review* **22** (4), pp. 12–15.

Anderson C, Deepak B V, Amoateng-Adjepong Y and Zarich S (2005) Benefits of comprehensive inpatient education and discharge planning combined with outpatient support in elderly patients with congestive heart failure. *Congestive Heart Failure* **11** (6), pp. 315–321.

Anderson M K, Markenvard J D, Schjott H, Nielson H L and Gustafason F (2005) Effects of a nurse-based heart failure clinic on drug utilization and admissions in a community hospital setting. *Scandinavian Cardiovascular Journal* **39** (4), pp. 199–205.

Andrew P (2003) Diastolic heart failure demystified. *Chest* **124** (2), pp. 744–753.

Appleton B (2004) The role of exercise training in patients with chronic heart failure. *British Journal of Nursing* **13** (8), pp. 452–456.

Aquilar D, Skali H, Moye L A, Lewis E F, Gaziano J M, Rutherford J D et al. (2004) Alcohol consumption and prognosis in patients with left ventricular systolic dysfunction after a myocardial infarction. *Journal of the American College of Cardiology* **43** (11), pp. 2015–2021.

Austin J, Williams R, Linda R, Moseley L and Hutchinson S (2005) Randomised controlled trial of cardiac rehabilitation in elderly patients with heart failure. *European Journal of Heart Failure* **7** (3), pp. 411–417.

Azevedo C F, Cheng S and Lima J A (2005) Cardiac imaging to identify patients at risk for developing heart failure after myocardial infarction. *Current Heart Failure Reports* **2** (4), pp. 183–188.

Badgett R G, Lucey C R and Mulrow C D (1997) Can the clinical examination diagnose left-sided heart failure in adults? *Journal of the American Medical Association* **277** (21), pp. 1712–1719.

Baig M K, Mahon N, McKenna W J, Caforio A L P, Bonow R O, Francis G S et al. (1999) The pathophysiology of advanced heart failure. *Heart and Lung* **28** (2), pp. 87–97.

Bardy G H, Lee K L, Mark D B, Poole J E, Packer D L, Boineau R et al. (2005) Amiodarone or an implantable cardioverter-defibrillator for congestive heart failure. *The New England Journal of Medicine* **352** (20), pp. 225–237.

Barnes S, Gott M and Payne S (2006) Communication in heart failure: perspectives from older people and primary care professionals. *Health & Social Care in the Community* **14** (6), pp. 482–490.

Barry W L and Sarembock I J (1998) Cardiogenic shock: therapy and prevention. *Clinical Cardiology* **21** (2), pp. 72–80.

Bartenek J, Vanderheyden M, Wijns W, Timmermans F, Vanderkerkhove B, Villa A et al. (2007) Bone marrow derived cells for cardiac stem cell therapy: safe or still under scrutiny? Nature Clinical Practice. *Cardiovascular Medicine* **4** (S1), pp. 100–105.

Baxter A J, Spensley A, Hildreth A, Karimova G, O'Connell J E and Gray C S (2002) Beta-blockers in older persons with heart failure: tolerability and impact on quality of life. *Heart* **88** (6), pp. 611–614.

Bell D S H (2002) Diabetic cardiomyopathy: a unique entity or a complication of coronary artery disease? *Diabetes Care* **18** (5), pp. 708–714.

Bell D S H (2003) Heart failure: the frequent, forgotten, and often fatal complication of diabetes. *Diabetes Care* **26** (8), pp. 2433–2441.

Bellardinelli R, Georgiou D, Cianci G and Purcaro A (1999) Randomised controlled trial of long term moderate exercise training in chronic heart failure: effects on functional capacity, quality of life, and clinical outcome. *Circulation* **99** (9), pp. 1173–1182.

Beniaminovitz A, Lang C C, LaManca J and Mancini D (2002) Selective low leg muscle training alleviates dyspnoea in patients with heart failure. *Journal of the American College of Cardiology* **40** (9), pp. 1602–1608.

Bertoni A G, Goff D C, D'Agnostino R B, Liu K, Hundley W G, Lima J A et al. (2006) Diabetic cardiomyopathy and sub clinical cardiovascular disease: the Multi-Ethnic Study of Atherosclerosis (MESA). *Diabetes Care* **29** (3), pp. 588–594.

Bessen H A (1986) Therapeutic and toxic effects of digitalis: William Withering, 1785. *The Journal of Emergency Medicine* **4** (3), pp. 243–248.

Blue L, Lang E, McMurray J J V, Davie A P, McDonagh T A, Murdoch D R et al. (2001) Randomised controlled trial of specialist nurse intervention in heart failure. *British Medical Journal* **323** (7315), pp. 715–718.

Bozkurt B and Deswal A (2005) Obesity as a prognostic factor in chronic symptomatic heart failure. *American Heart Journal* **150** (6), pp. 1233–1239.

British Cardiac Society, British Hypertension Society, Diabetes UK, HEART UK, Primary Care Cardiovascular Society, Stroke Association (2005) JBS 2: Joint British Societies' guidelines on prevention of cardiovascular disease in clinical practice. *Heart* **91** Supplement 5, pp. v1–52.

Brophy J M, Joseph L and Rouleau J L (2001) Beta-blockers in congestive heart failure. A Bayesian meta-analysis. *Annals of Internal Medicine*, **134**, (7), pp. 550–560.

Bryson C L, Mukamal K J, Mittleman M A, Fried L P, Hirsch C H, Kitzman D W et al. (2006) The association of alcohol consumption and incident heart failure: the Cardiovascular Health Study. *Journal of the American College of Cardiology* **48** (2), pp. 305–311.

Buetow S A and Coster G D (2001) Do general practice patients with heart failure understand its nature and seriousness, and want improved information? *Patient Education and Counseling* **45** (3), pp. 181–185.

Buetow S A, Goodyear S F and Coster G (2001) Coping strategies in the self-management of chronic heart failure. *Family Practice* **18** (2), pp. 117–122.

Bungard T J, McAlister F A, Johnson J A and Tsuyuki R T (2001) Underutilisation of ACE inhibitors in patients with congestive heart failure. *Drugs* **61** (14), pp. 2021–2033.

Burian J, Buser P and Eriksson U (2005) Myocarditis: the immunologists view on pathogenesis and treatment. *Swiss Medical Weekly* **135** (25–26), pp. 359–364.

Buxton A E, Lee K L, Fisher J D, Josephson M E, Prystowsky E N and Hafley G (1999) A randomized study of the prevention of sudden death in patients with coronary artery disease. Multicenter Unsustained Tachycardia Trial Investigators. *The New England Journal of Medicine* **341** (25), pp. 1882–1890.

Caldwell M A, Peters K J and Dracup K S (2005) A simplified education program improves knowledge, self care behaviour, and disease severity in heart failure patients in rural settings. *American Heart Journal* **150** (5), pp. 983.

Calvert M J, Freemantle N, Yao G, Cleland J G F, Billingham L and Daubert J et al. (2005) Cost-effectiveness of cardiac resynchronization therapy: results from the CARE-HF trial. *European Heart Journal*, **26** (24), pp. 681–688.

Chambers J, Fuat A, Liddiard S, McDonagh T, Monaghan M, Nihoyannopoulus P et al. (2004) Community echocardiography for heart failure: a consensus statement from representatives of the British Society of Echocardiography, the British Heart Failure Society, the Coronary Heart Disease Collaborative and the Primary Care Cardiovascular Society. *British Journal of Cardiology* **11** (5), pp. 399–402.

Chinnaiyan K M, Alexander D, Maddens M and McCullough P A (2007) Curriculum in cardiology: Integrated diagnosis and management of diastolic heart failure. *American Heart Journal* **153** (2), pp. 189–200.

Chow A W C, Lane R E and Cowie M R (2003) New pacing technologies for heart failure. *British Medical Journal* **326** (7398), pp. 1073–1077.

Cintron G, Bigas C, Linares E, Aranda J M and Hernandez E (1983) Nurse practitioner role in chronic congestive heart failure clinic: in hospital time, costs, and patient satisfaction. *Heart and Lung* **12** (3), pp. 237–240.

Clark A and Nadash P (2004) The effectiveness of a nurse-led transitional care model for patients with congestive heart failure. *Home Healthcare Nurse* **22** (3), pp. 160–162.

Clark A L and Coats A J S (2000) Unreliability of cardiothoracic ratio as a marker of left ventricular impairment: Comparison with radionuclide ventriculography and echocardiography. *Postgraduate Medical Journal* **76** (895), pp. 289–291.

Clarke K W, Gray D and Hampton J R (1995) How common is heart failure? Evidence from PACT (prescribing analysis and cost) data in Nottingham. *Journal of Public Health Medicine* **17** (4), pp. 459–464.

Clegg A J, Scott D A, Loveman E, Colquitt J, Hutchinson J, Royle P et al (2005) The clinical and cost effectiveness of left ventricular assist devices for end stage heart failure: a systematic review and economic evaluation. *Health Technology Assessment* **9** (45), pp. 1–148.

Cleland J G, Daubert J C, Erdmann E, Freemantle N, Gras D, Kappenberger L et al. (2005) The effect of cardiac resynchronization on morbidity and mortality in heart failure. Cardiac Resynchronisation-Heart Failure (CARE-HF) Study Investigators. *The New England Journal of Medicine* **352** (15), pp. 1539–1549.

Coats A J S (2001) What causes the symptoms of heart failure? *Heart* **86** (5), pp. 574–578.

Coats A J S, Adamopoulus S, Radelli A, McCanca A, Meyer T E and Berbadi L (1992) Controlled trial of physical training in heart failure. *Circulation* **85** (6), pp. 2119–2131.

Cody R J, Kubo S H and Pickworth K K (1994) Diuretic treatment for the sodium retention of congestive heart failure. *Archives of Internal Medicine* **154** (17), pp. 1905–1914.

Cody R J and Pickworth K K (1994) Approaches to diuretic therapy and electrolyte imbalance in congestive heart failure. *Cardiology Clinics* **12** (1), pp. 37–50.

Cohn J N and Tognoni G (2001) Randomised trial of the angiotensin receptor blocker valsartan in chronic heart failure. The Valsartan Heart Failure Trial Investigators. *The New England Journal of Medicine* **345** (23), pp. 1667–1675.

Collins S D, Baffour R and Waksmans R (2007) Cell therapy in myocardial infarction. *Cardiovascular Revascularisation Medicine: including Molecular Interventions* **8** (1), pp. 43–51.

Colucci W S, Packer M, Bristow M R, Gilbert E M, Cohn J N, Fowler M B et al. (1996) Carvedilol inhibits clinical progression in patients with mild symptoms of heart failure. US Carvedilol Heart Failure Study Group. *Circulation* **94** (11), pp. 2800–2806.

Connolly M J, Crowley J J and Vestral R E (1992) Clinical significance of crepitations in elderly patients following acute hospital admission: a prospective study. *Age and Aging* **21** (1), pp. 43–8.

Connolly S J, Hallstrom A P, Cappato R, Schron E B, Kuck K H, Zipes D P et al. (2000a) Meta-analysis of the implantable cardioverter defibrillator secondary prevention trials. AVID, CASH and CIDS studies. Antiarrhythmics vs Implantable Defibrillator Study. Cardiac Arrest Study Hamburg. Canadian Implantable Defibrillator Study. *European Heart Journal* **21** (24), pp. 2071–2078.

Connolly S J, Gent M, Roberts R S, Doarian P, Roy D, Sheldon R S, et al. (2000b) Canadian implantable defibrillator study (CIDS): a randomized trial of the implantable cardioverter defibrillator against amiodarone. *Circulation* **101** (11), pp. 1297–1302.

Constanzo M R, Guglin M, Saltzberg M T, Jessup M L, Bart B A, Teerlink J R, et al (2007) Ultrafiltration versus intravenous diuretics for patients hospitalised for acute decompensated heart failure. *Journal of the American College of Cardiology* **49** (6), pp. 675–683.

Cook D J (1990) Clinical assessment of central venous pressure in the critically ill. *The American Journal of Medical Sciences* **299** (3), pp. 175–178.

Cooper H A, Exner D V and Domanski, M J (2000) Light to moderate alcohol consumption and prognosis in patients with left ventricular systolic dysfunction. *Journal of the American College of Cardiology* **35** (7), pp. 1753–1759.

Coviello J S and Nystrom K V (2003) Obesity and heart failure. *The Journal of Cardiovascular Nursing* **18** (5), pp. 360–366.

Cowie M R and Kirby M (2003) *Managing heart failure in primary care: a practical guide.* Chipping Norton: Bladon Medical Publishing.

Cowie M R, Struthers A D, Wood D A, Coats A J S, Thompson S G, Pole-Wilson P A and Sutton G C (1997) Value of natriuretic peptides in assessment of patients with possible new heart failure in primary care. *The Lancet* **350** (9088), pp. 1349–1352.

Cowie M R, Wood D A, Coats A J S, Thompson S G, Poole-Wilson P A, Suresh V et al. (1999) Incidence and aetiology of heart failure: a population-based study. *European Heart Journal* **20** (6), pp. 421–428.

Cowie M R, Wood D A, Coats A J S, Thompson S G, Suresh V, Poole-Wilson P A et al. (2000) Survival of patients with a new diagnosis of heart failure: a population based study. *Heart* **83** (5), pp. 505–510.

Crawford P and Hendry A (1997) Investigation of left ventricular dysfunction in acute dyspnoea. *British Medical Journal* **314** (7085), pp. 936–940.

Curtis J P, Selter J G, Wang Y, Rathore, S S, Jovin I S, Jadbabaie F et al. (2005) The obesity paradox: body mass index and outcomes in patients with heart failure. *Archives of Internal Medicine* **165** (1), pp. 55–61.

Davenport C, Cheng E Y L, Kwok Y T T, Lai A H O, Wakabayashi T, Hyde C et al. (2006) Assessing the diagnostic test accuracy of natriuretic peptides and ECG in the diagnosis of left ventricular systolic dysfunction: a systematic review and meta-analysis. *The British Journal of General Practice* **56** (522), pp. 48–56.

Davie A P and McMurray J (1997) Investigation of left ventricular dysfunction in acute dyspnoea. A 100% sensitivity would be difficult to achieve. *British Medical Journal Letters* **315** (7108), p. 604.

Davie A P, Francis C M, Love M P, Caruna L, Starkey I R, Shaw T R D et al (1996a) Value of the electrocardiogram in identifying heart failure due to left ventricular systolic dysfunction. *British Medical Journal* **312** (7025), pp. 222–225.

Davie A P, Love M P and MacMurray J J V (1996b) Value of the electrocardigram in identifying heart failure due to left ventricular systolic dysfunction. *British Medical Journal* **313** (7052), pp.300–301.

Davies M K, Hobbs F D R, Davis R C, Kenkre J E, Roalfe A K, Hare R et al. (2001) Prevalence of left-ventricular systolic dysfunction and heart failure in the echocardiographic heart of England screening study: a population based study. *The Lancet* **358** (9280), pp. 439–444.

Davis R C, Hobbs F D R and Lip G Y H (2000) ABC of heart failure: history and epidemiology. *British Medical Journal* **320** (7226), pp. 39–42.

Davison R and Cannon R (1974) Estimation of central venous pressure by examination of jugular veins. *American Heart Journal* **87** (3), pp. 279–282.

Davos C H, Doehner W, Rauchhaus M, Cicoira M, Francis D P, Coats A J S et al. (2003) Body mass index and survival in patients with chronic heart failure without cachexia; the importance of obesity. *Journal of Cardiac Failure* **9** (1), pp 29–35.

Dawn B, Zuba-Surma E K, Abdel-Latif A, Tiwari S and Bolli R (2005) Cardiac stem cell therapy for myocardial regeneration: a clinical perspective. *Minerva Cardioangiologica Europa* **53** (6), pp. 549–564.

DeBusk R, Drory Y and Goldstein I et al. (2000) Management of sexual dysfunction in patients with cardiovascular disease: recommendations of the Princeton Consensus Panel. *American Journal of Cardiology* **86** (2), pp. 175–181.

Demopoulus L, Yeh M and Gentilucci M (1997) Non-selective beta-adrenergic blockade with carvedilol does not hinder the benefits of exercise training in patients with congestive heart failure. *Circulation* **95** (7), pp. 1764–1767.

Department of Health (2000a) *The NHS Plan*. London: HMSO.

Department of Health (2000b) *National Service Framework for Coronary Heart Disease*. London: HMSO.

Department of Health (2003) *Developing Services for Heart Failure*. London: HMSO.

Dincer H E and O'Neill W (2005) Deleterious effects of sleep disordered breathing on the heart and vascular system. *Respiration* **73** (1), pp. 124–130.

Djousse L, Levy D, Benjamin E J, Blease S J, Russ A, Alrson M G et al. (2004) Long-term alcohol consumption and the risk of atrial fibrillation in the Framingham Study. *The American Journal of Cardiology* 93 (6), pp. 710–713.

Doust J A, Pietrzak E, Dobson A and Glasziou P P (2005) How well does B-type natriuretic peptide predict death and cardiac events in patients with heart failure: systematic review. *British Medical Journal* **330** (7492), p. 625

Doval H C, Nul D R, Grancelli H O, Perrone S V, Bortman G R and Curiel R (1994) Randomised trial of low-dose amiodarone in severe congestive heart failure. Grupo de Estudio de la Sobrevida en la Insuficiencia Cardiaca en Argentina (GESICA). *The Lancet* **344** (8921), pp. 493–498.

Doyle J J, Neugut A I, Jacobsen J S, Grann V R and Hershman D L (2005) Chemotherapy and cardiotoxicity in older breast cancer patients; a population based study. *Journal of Clinical Oncology* **23** (34), pp. 8597–8605.

Drazner J H, Rame J E and Dries D L (2003) Third heart sound and elevated jugular venous pressure as markers of the subsequent development of heart failure in patients with asymptomatic left ventricular dysfunction. *American Journal of Medicine* 114 (6), pp. 499–500.

Dubrey S W, Cha K, Skinner M, LaValley M and Falk R H (1997) Familial and primary (AL) cardiac amyloidosis: echocardiographically similar disease with distinctly different clinical outcomes. *Heart* **78** (1), pp. 74–82.

Eilen S D, Crawford M H and O'Rourke R A (1983) Accuracy of precordial palpitation for detecting increased left ventricular volume. *Annals of Internal Medicine* **99** (5), pp. 628–630.

Elhendy A, Sozzi F, Van Domburg R T, Bax J J, Schinkel A F L, Roelandt J R T C et al. (2005) Effect of myocardial ischemia during dobutamine stress echocardiography on cardiac mortality in patients with heart failure secondary to ischaemic cardiomyopathy. *American Journal of Cardiology* 96 (4), pp. 469–473.

Elkayam U, Tasissa G, Binanay C, Stevenson L W, Gheorghiade M, Warnica J W et al. (2007) Use and impact of inotropes and vasodilator therapy in hospitalised patients with severe heart failure. *American Heart Journal* **153** (1), pp. 98–104.

Erbs S, Linke A, Gielen S, Fiehn E, Walther C, Yu J et al. (2003) Exercise training in patients with severe chronic heart failure: impact on left ventricular performance and cardiac size. A retrospective analysis of the Leipzig Heart Failure Training Trial. *European Journal of Cardiovascular Prevention and Rehabilitation* **10** (5), pp. 336–344.

Erbs S, Linke A and Hambrecht R (2006) Effects of exercise training on mortality in patients with coronary heart disease. *Coronary Artery Disease* **17** (3), pp. 219–225.

Erickson V S, Westlake C A, Dracup K A, Woo M A and Hage A (2003) Sleep disturbance symptoms in patients with heart failure. *AACN Clinical Issues: Advanced Practice in Acute and Critical Care* **14** (4), pp. 477–487.

Evangelista L S and Miller P S (2006) Overweight and obesity in the context of heart failure: implications for practise and future research. *Journal of Cardiovascular Nursing* **21** (1), pp. 27–33.

Evangelista L S, Doering L V and Dracup K (2000) Usefulness of a history of tobacco and alcohol use in predicting multiple heart failure admission among veterans. *The American Journal of Cardiology* **86** (12), pp. 1339–1342.

Fabrizio L and Regan T J (1994) Alcoholic cardiomyopathy. *cardiovascular Drugs and Therapy* **8** (1), pp. 89–94.

Faris R, Falther M, Purcell H, Pole-Wilson P and Coats A (2006) Diuretics for heart failure. *Cochrane Database of Systematic Reviews* (1).

Feldman A M, de Lissovoy G, Bristow M R, Saxon L A, De Marco T, Kass D A et al. (2005) Cost effectiveness of cardiac resynchronization therapy in the Comparison of Medical Therapy, Pacing, and Defibrillation in Heart Failure (COMPANION) trial. *Journal of the American College of Cardiology* **46** (12), pp. 2311–2321.

Fleg J L (2002) Can exercise conditioning be effective in older heart failure patients? *Heart Failure Reviews* **7** (1), pp. 99–103.

Floras J S (2005) Sleep apnoea in heart failure: implications of sympathetic nervous system activation for disease progression and treatment. *Current Heart Failure Reports* **2** (4), pp. 212–217.

Flynn K J, Powell L H, Mendes de Leon C F, Munoz R, Eaton C B, Downs D L et al. (2005). Increasing self management skills in heart failure patients: a pilot study. *Congestive Heart Failure* **11** (6), pp. 297–302.

Fonseca C, Mota T, Morais H, Matias F, Costa C, Oliveira A G et al. (2004) The value of the electrocardiogram and chest X-ray for confirming or refuting a suspected diagnosis of heart failure in the community. *European Journal of Heart Failure* **6** (6), pp. 807–812.

Fox K (2004) Accreditation in community echocardiography. *British Journal of Cardiology* **11** (5), p. 402.

Frazier O H (2003) Ventricular assist devices and total artificial hearts: a historical perspective. *Cardiology Clinics* **21** (1), pp. 1–13.

French B A (1998) Gene therapy and cardiovascular disease. *Current Opinions in Cardiology* **13** (3), pp. 205–213.

Fried T, van Doorn C, O'Leary J, Tinetti M and Drickamer M (1999) Older persons preferences for site of terminal care. *Annals of Internal Medicine* **131** (2), pp. 109–112.

Friedmann E, Thomas S A, Liu F, Morton P G, Chapa D and Gottlieb S S (2006) Relationship of depression, anxiety, and social isolation to chronic heart failure outpatient mortality. *American Heart Journal* **152** (5), p. 940.

Fuat A, Hungin A P S and Murphy J J (2003) Barriers to accurate diagnosis and effective management of heart failure in primary care: qualitative study. *British Medical Journal* **326** (7382), p. 196.

Galatius S, Gustafsson F, Atar D and Hildebrandt P R (2004) Tolerability of beta-blocker initiation and titration with bisoprolol and carvedilol in congestive heart failure – a randomized comparison. *Cardiology* **102** (3), pp. 160–165.

Gasparini M, Regoli F, Galimberti P, Ceriotti C, Bonadies M, Mangiavacchi M et al. (2007) Three years of cardiac resynchronisation therapy: could superior benefits be obtained in patients with heart failure and narrow QRS? *Pacing and Clinical Electrophysiology* **S1** S34–39.

Gerecht N S and Itskovitz E J (2004) Human embryonic stem cells: a potential source for cellular therapy. *American Journal of Transplantation* **4** (S6), pp. 51–57.

Gertz M A, Lacy M Q and Dispenzieri A (2005) Amyloidosis: recognition, confirmation, prognosis and therapy. *Mayo Clinic Proceedings* **74** (5), pp. 490–494.

GESICA Investigators (2005) Randomised trial of telephone intervention in chronic heart failure: DIAL trial. *British Medical Journal* **331** (7514), p. 425.

Ghani J K, Kadakia S, Cooper R et al. (1988) Precipitating factors leading to decompensation in heart failure: traits among urban blacks. *Archives of Internal Medicine* **148** (9), pp. 2013–2016.

Gheorghiade M, Abraham W T, Albert N M, Gattis-Stough W, Greenberg B H, O'Conner C M, et al. (2007) Relationship between admission serum sodium concentration and clinical outcomes in patients hospitalised for heart failure: an analysis from the OPTIMIZE-HF registry. *European Heart Journal*, Advance Access published online on 19 February 2007.

Giannuzzi, P (2003) Antiremodeling effect of long-term exercise training in patients with stable chronic heart failure: results of the Exercise in Left Ventricular Dysfunction and Chronic Heart Failure (ELVD-CHF) Trial. *Circulation* **108** (5) pp. 554–559.

Gibbs L M E, Hatri A K and Gibbs J S R (2006) Survey of specialist palliative care and heart failure: September 2004. *Palliative Medicine* **20** (6), pp. 603–609.

Gillespie N D, McNeil G, Pringle T, Ogston S, Struthers A D and Pringle S D (1997) Cross sectional study of the contribution of clinical assessment and simple cardiac investigations to the diagnosis of left ventricular systolic function in patients with acute dyspnoea. *British Medical Journal* **314** (7085), pp. 936–940.

Gold L D and Krumholz H M (2006) Gender differences in treatment of heart failure and acute myocardial infarction: a question of quality or epidemiology? *Cardiology in Review* **14** (4), pp. 180–186.

Goldstein S (2004) The changing epidemiology of sudden death in heart failure. *Current Heart Failure Reports* **1** (3), pp. 93–97.

Good C B, McDermott L and McCloskey B (1995) Diet and serum potassium in patients on ACE inhibitors. *Journal of the American Medical Association* **274** (7), p. 538.

Gustafsson I, Torp-Pederson C, Kober L, Gustafsson F and Hilberant P (1999) Effect of the angiotensin-converting enzyme inhibitor trandolapril on mortality and morbidity in diabetic patients with left ventricular dysfunction after acute myocardial infarction. Trace Study Group. *Journal of the American College of Cardiology* **34** (1), pp. 83–89.

Gwadry-Sridhar F H, Arnold J M, Zhang Y, Brown J E, Marchiori G and Guyatt G (2005) Pilot study to determine the impact of a multidisciplinary educational intervention in patients hospitalised with heart failure. *American Heart Journal* **150** (5), pp. 982–989.

Gwinnutt C L, Columb M and Harris R (2000) Outcome after cardiac arrest in adults in UK hospitals: effect of the 1997 guidelines. *Resuscitation* **47** (2), pp. 125–135.

Hall J A, French T K, Rasmusson K D, Vesty J C, Roberts C A, Rimmasch H L et al. (2005) The paradox of obesity in patients with heart failure. *Journal of the American Academy of Nurse Practitioners* **17** (12), pp. 542–546.

Hambleton M, Hahn H, Pleger S T, Kuhn M C, Klevitsky R, Carr A N et al. (2006) Pharmaceutical and gene based inhibition of protein kinase $C^{\alpha\beta}$ enhances cardiac contractility and attenuates heart failure. *Circulation* **114** (6), pp. 574–582.

Hambrecht R, Fiehn E and Neibaier J (1997) Effects of endurance training on mitochondrial ultrastructure and fibre type distribution in skeletal muscles of patients with stable chronic heart failure. *Journal of the American College of Cardiology* **29** (5), pp. 527–537.

Hamner J B and Ellison K J (2005) Predictors of hospital readmission after discharge in patients with congestive heart failure. *Heart and Lung* **34** (4), pp. 231–239.

Hanumanthu S, Butler J, Chomsky D et al (1997) Effect of heart failure program on hospitalisation frequency and exercise tolerance. *Circulation* **96** (9), pp. 2842–2848.

Harlan W R (1977) Chronic congestive heart failure in coronary artery disease: clinical criteria. *Annals of Internal Medicine* **86** (2), pp. 133–138.

Harrison M B, Browne G B, Roberts J, Tugwell P, Gafni A and Graham I D (2002) Quality of life of individuals with heart failure: a randomized trial of the effectiveness of two models of hospital-to-home transition. *Medical Care* **40** (4), pp. 271–282.

Hill E E, Herijgers P, Claus P, Vanderschueren S, Herregods M C and Peetermans W E (2007) Infective endocarditis: changing epidemiology and predictors of 6-month mortality: a prospective cohort study. *European Heart Journal* **28** (2), pp. 196–203.

Hobbs F D (2000) Management of heart failure: evidence versus practice. Does current prescribing provide optimal treatment for heart failure patients? *The British Journal of General Practice* **50** (458), pp. 735–42.

Holland R, Battersby J, Harvey I, Lenaghen E, Smith J and Hay L (2005) Systematic review of multidisciplinary interventions in heart failure. *Heart* **91** (7), pp. 899–906.

Hooley P J, Butler G and Howlett J G (2005) The relationship of quality of life, depression, and caregiver burden in outpatients with congestive heart failure. *Congestive Heart Failure* **11** (6), pp. 303–310.

Houghton A R, Sparrow N J, Toms E and Cowley A J (1997) Should general practitioners use the electrocardiogram to select patients with suspected heart failure for echocardiography? *International Journal of Cardiology* **62** (1), pp. 31–36.

Hunt S A, Baker D W, Chin M H, Cinquegrani M P, Feldman A M, Francis G S et al. (2001) *ACC/AHA Guidelines for the Evaluation and Management of Chronic Heart Failure in the Adult.* Bethseda: American College of Cardiology.

Ismail A A, Wing S, Ferguson J, Hutchinson T A, Magder, S and Flegel K M (1987) Interobserver agreement by auscultation in the presence of a third heart sound in patients with congestive heart failure. *Chest* **91** (6), pp. 870–3.

Jaarsma T and Dracup K (2001) Determinisation of health care utilisation by patients with chronic heart failure. In Stewart S and Blue L, *Chronic Heart Failure: a Practical Guide to Specialist Nurse Intervention.* London: BMJ Books.

Jaarsama T, Stromberg A, De Geest S, Fridlund B, Heikkila J, Martensson J et al. (2006) Heart failure management programmes in Europe. *European Journal of Cardiovascular Nursing* **5** (3), pp. 197–205.

Jackson G, Gibbs C R, Davies M K and Lip, G Y (2000) ABC of heart failure: pathophysiology. *British Medical Journal* **320** (7228), pp. 167–170.

Jacob A J, McLaren K M and Boon N A (1991) Effects of abstinence on alcoholic heart muscle disease. *American Journal of Cardiology* **68** (8), pp. 805–807.

Januzzi J L, Van Kimmenade R, Lainchbury J, Bayes-Genis A, Ordonez-Llanos J, Santalo-Bel M et al. (2005) NT-proBNP testing for diagnosis and short term prognosis in acute destabilised heart failure: an international analysis of 1256 patients. *European Heart Journal* **27** (3), pp. 330–337.

Jessup M and Brozena S C (2003) Support devices for end stage heart failure. *Cardiology Clinics* **21** (1), pp. 135–139.

Joekes K, Elderen T van and Schreurs K (2007) Self-efficacy and overprotection are related to quality of life, psychological well-being and self-management in cardiac patients. *Journal of Health Psychology* **12** (1), pp. 4–16.

Jolly L (2002) The role of the specialist nurse. *Heart* **88** (SII), pp. ii33-ii35.

Joshi N (1999) The third heart sound. *Southern Medical Journal* **92** (8), pp. 756–61.

Jovicic A, Holroyd L J M and Straus S E (2006) Effects of self-management intervention on health outcomes of patients with heart failure: a systematic review of randomized controlled trials. *BMC Cardiovascular Disorders* **6** (1), pp. 43–51.

Juenger J, Schelberg D, Kraemer S, Haunstetter A, Zugck C, Herzog W et al. (2002) Health related quality of life in patients with congestive heart failure: comparison with other chronic diseases and relation to functional variables. *Heart* **87** (3), pp. 235–41.

Juurlink D N, Mamdani M M, Lee D S, Kopp A, Austin P C, Laupacis A et al. (2004) Rates of hyperkalemia after publication of the Randomized Aldactone Evaluation Study. *The New England Journal of Medicine* **351** (6), pp. 543–551.

Kamath S A, Meo N J D P, Canham R M, Uddin F, Toto K H, Nelson L L et al. (2006) Low voltage on the electrocardiogram is a marker of disease severity and a risk factor for adverse outcomes in patients with heart failure due to systolic dysfunction. *American Heart Journal* **152** (2), pp. 355–361.

Kannel W B and Belanger A J (1991) Epidemiology of heart failure. *American Heart Journal* **121** (3), pp. 951–957.

Kannel W B (2000) Incidence and epidemiology of heart failure. *Heart Failure Reviews* **5** (2), pp. 167–173.

Kareti K R, Chiong J R, Hsu S S and Miller A B (2005) Congestive heart failure and atrial fibrillation: rhythm versus rate control. *Journal of Cardiac Failure* **11** (3), pp. 164–172.

Kellerman J J, Shemesh J and Ben-Ari E (1988) Contraindications to physical training in patients with impaired ventricular function. *European Heart Journal* **9** Supplement F, pp. 71–76.

Kenchaiah S, Evans J C, Levy D, Wilson P W, Benjamin E J, Larson M G et al. (2002) Obesity and the risk of heart failure. *The New England Journal of Medicine* **347** (5), pp. 303–313.

Kernan W N, Castellsague J, Perlman G D and Ostfeld A (1994) Incidence of hospitalization for digitalis toxicity among elderly Americans. *The American Journal of Medicine* **96** (5), pp. 426–431.

Kervio G, Ville N S, Leclercq C, Daubert J C and Carre F (2004) Intensity and daily reliability of the six-minute walk test in moderate chronic heart failure patients. *Archives of Physical Medicine and Rehabilitation* **85** (9), pp.1513–1518.

Khan N A, Ma I, Thompson C R, Humphries K, Salem D N, Sarnak M J and Levin A (2005) Kidney function and mortality among patients with left ventricular systolic dysfunction. *Journal of the American Society of Nephrology* **17** (1), pp. 244–253.

Kjekshus J, Swedberg K and Sanpinn S (1992) Effects on enalapril on long term mortality in severe congestive heart failure. CONSENSUS Trial Group. *American Journal of Cardiology* **69** (1), pp. 103–107.

Klatsky A L, Chartier D, Udaltsova N, Gronningen S, Brar S, Freidman G D and Lundstrom R J (2005) Alcohol drinking and risk of hospitalisation for heart failure with and without associated coronary artery disease. *The American Journal of Cardiology* **96** (3), pp.346–351.

Konstam M A, Neaton J D, Poole-Wilson P A, Pitt B, Segal R, Sharma D et al. (2005) Comparison of losartan and captopril on heart failure-related outcomes and symptoms from the losartan heart failure survival study (ELITE II). *American Heart Journal* **150** (1), pp. 123–131.

Kornowski R, Zeeli D, Averbach M (1995) Intensive home surveillance prevents hospitalisation and improves morbidity rates among elderly patients with severe congestive heart failure. *American Heart Journal* **129** (4), pp. 762–766.

Krantrowitz A, Tjonneland S, Freed P S, Philips S J, Butner A N and Sherman J N Jnr. (1968) Initial clinical experience with intraaortic balloon pumping in cardiogenic shock. *Journal of the American Medical Association* **203** (2), pp. 113–118.

Kuck K H, Cappato R, Siebels J and Ruppel R (2000) Randomized comparison of antiarrythmic drug therapy with implantable defibrillators in patients resuscitated from cardiac arrest: the Cardiac Arrest Study Hamburg (CASH). *Circulation* **102** (7), pp. 748–754.

Lackey J (2004) Cognitive impairment and congestive heart failure. *Nursing Standard* **18** (44), pp. 33–36.

Lakka H M, Lakka T A, Tuomilehto J and Salomnen J T (2002) Abdominal obesity is associated with increased risk of acute coronary events in men. *European Heart Journal* **23** (9), pp. 706–713.

Lampert M B and Lang R M (1995) Peripartum cardiomyopathy. *American Heart Journal* **130** (4), pp. 860–870.

Latour-Perez J, Covesorts F J, Abad-Terrado C, Abraira V and Zamora J (2005) Accuracy of B-type natriuretic peptide levels in the diagnosis of left ventricular dysfunction and heart failure: a systematic review. *European Journal of Heart Failure* **8** (4), pp. 390–399.

Lauer M S, Anderson K M, Kannel W B and Levy D (1991) The impact of obesity on left ventricular mass and geometry: the Framingham Heart Study. *Journal of the American Medical Association* **266** (2), pp. 231–236.

Lee W K and Regan T J (2002) Alcoholic cardiomyopathy: is it dose dependent? *Congestive Heart Failure* **8** (6), pp. 303–6.

Lemola K, Brunckhorst C, Helfenstein U, Oeschslin E, Jenni R and Duru F (2005) Predictors of adverse outcome in patients with arrythmogenic right ventricular dysplasia/cardiomyopathy: long term experience of a tertiary centre. *Heart* **91** (9), pp. 1167–1172.

Leslie S J, Emmanuel Y, Francis C M and Flapan A D (2004) The treatment of peripartum cardiomyopathy. *British Journal of Cardiology* **11** (5), pp. 393–396.

Levick J R (1995) *An Introduction to Cardiovascular Physiology,* 2nd Edition, Oxford: Butterworth-Heinemann.

Lightwood J M and Glantz S A (1997) Short term economic and health benefits of smoking cessation: myocardial infarction and stroke. *Circulation* **96** (4), pp. 1089–1096.

Linde C, Braunschweig F, Gadler F, Bailleul C and Daubert J C (2003) Long-term improvements in quality of life by biventricular pacing in patients with chronic heart failure: results from the Multisite Stimulation in Cardiomyopathy study (MUSTIC). *The American Journal of Cardiology* **91** (9), pp. 1090–1095.

Lipiecki J, Durel N and Ponsonnaille J (2006) Which patients with ischaemic heart disease could benefit from cell replacement therapy? *European Heart Journal* **8** Supplement, H3–7.

Lloyd-Williams F, Mair F S and Leitner, M (2002) Exercise training and heart failure: a systematic review of current evidence. *British Journal of General Practice* **52** (474), pp. 47–55.

Lloyd-Williams F, Beaton S, Goldstein P, Mair F, May C and Capewell S (2005) Patients' and nurses' views of nurse-led heart failure clinics in general practice: a qualitative study. *Chronic Illness* **1** (1), pp. 39–47.

Lyratzopoulos G, Cook G A, McElduff P, Havely D, Edwards R and Heller R F (2004) Assessing the impact of heart failure specialist services on patient populations. *BMC Health Services Research* **4** (1), p. 10.

Madsen B K, Videbaek R, Stokholm H M, Mortensen L S and Hansen J F (1996) Prognostic value of echocardiography in 190 patients with chronic congestive heart failure: a comparison with New York Heart Association functional classes and radionuclide ventriculography. *Cardiology* **87** (3), p. 250–256.

Mahmudi M, McDonagh S, Poole-Wilson P A and Dubrey S W (2003) Obstacles to the initiation of beta-blockers for heart failure in a specialised clinic within a district general hospital. *Heart* **89** (4), pp. 422–444.

Mair F S, Crowley T S and Bundred P E (1996) Prevalence, aetiology and management of heart failure in general practice. *The British Journal of General Practice* **46** (403), pp. 77–79.

Malki Q, Sharma N D, Afzal A, Ananthsubramaniam K, Abbas A, Jacobson G and Jafri S (2002) Clinical presentation, hospital length of stay, and readmission rate in patients with heart failure with preserved and decreased left ventricular systolic function. *Clinical Cardiology* **25** (4), pp. 149–152.

Mancini D M, Walter G, Reichek N, Lenkinski R, McCully R, Mullen J L and Wilson J R (1992) Contribution of skeletal muscle atrophy to exercise intolerance and altered muscle metabolism in heart failure. *Circulation* **85** (4), pp. 1364–1373.

Marcus F, Towbin J A, Zareba W, Moss A, Calkins H, Brown M and Gear K (2003) Arrhythmogenic right ventricular dysplasia/cardiomyopathy (ARVD/C): a multidisciplinary study: design and protocol. *Circulation* **107** (23), pp. 2975–2978.

Mariotti R, Castrogiovanni F, Becherini F, Cortese B, Rondini L and Mariani M (2004) Obesity, weight loss and heart failure. *European Heart Journal* Supplement **6** (6), F87–90.

Maron B J, Towbin J A, Thiene G, Antzelevitch C, Corrado D, Arnett D et al. (2006) Contemporary definitions and classification of the cardiomyopathies: an American Heart Association Scientific Statement from the Council on Clinical Cardiology, Heart Failure and Transplantation Committee; Quality of Care and Outcomes research and Functional Genomics and Transitional Biology Interdisciplinary Working Group; and Council on Epidemiology and Prevention. *Circulation* **113** (14), pp. 1807–1816.

Martensson J, Stromberg A, Dahlstrom U, Karlsson J E and Fridlund B (2005) Patients with heart failure in primary health care: effects of a nurse-led intervention on health-related quality of life and depression. *European Journal of Heart Failure* **7** (3), pp. 393–403.

Massie B M (2002) Obesity and heart failure – risk factor or mechanism? *The New England Journal of Medicine* **347** (5), pp. 358–360.

Masson S, Latini R, Anand I S, Vago T, Angelici L, Barlera S et al. (2006) Direct comparison of B-type natriuretic peptide (BNP) and amino-terminal proBNP in a large population of patients with chronic and symptomatic heart failure: the valsartan heart failure (Val-HeFT) data. *Clinical Chemistry* **52** (8), pp. 1528–1538.

Matsui Y, Fukada Y, Naito Y, Sasaki S and Yasuda, K (2005) A surgical approach to severe congestive heart failure – overlapping ventriculoplasty. *Journal of Cardiovascular Surgery* **20** (S6), S29–S34.

Mazza A, Tikhonoff V, Casiglia E and Pessina A C (2005) Predictors of congestive heart failure mortality in elderly people from the general population: The Cardiovascular Study in the Elderly (CASTEL). *International Heart Journal* **46** (3), pp. 419–431.

McAlister F A, Stewart S, Ferrua S and McMurray J J V (2004) Multidisciplinary strategies for the management of heart failure patients at high risk for admission. *Journal of the American College of Cardiology* **44** (4), pp. 810–819.

McCormick S A (1999) Advanced practice nursing for congestive heart failure. *Critical Care Nursing Quarterly* **21** (4), pp. 1–8.

McDonagh T A (2002) Screening for left ventricular dysfunction: a step too far? *Heart* **88** Supplement 2, pp. ii12–4.

McDonagh T A, Morrison C E, Lawrence A, Ford I, Tunstall-Pedoe H, McMurray J J and Dargie H J (1997) Symptomatic and asymptomatic left-ventricular systolic dysfunction in an urban population. *Lancet* **350** (9081), pp. 829–833.

McElvie R S, Teo K K, McCartney N, Humen D, Montague T and Yusuf S (1995) Effects of exercise training in patients with congestive heart failure: a critical review. *Journal of the American College of Cardiology* **25** (3), pp. 789–796.

McElvie R S, Yusuf S, Pericak D, Avezum A, Burns R J, Probstfield J et al. (1999) Comparison of candesartan, enalapril, and their combination in congestive heart failure: randomized evaluation of strategies for left ventricular dysfunction (RESOLVD) pilot study. The RESOLVD Pilot Study Investigators. *Circulation* **100** (10), pp. 1056–1064.

Mehta R and Feldman D (2005) Acute decompensated heart failure: best evidence and current practices. *Minerva Cardioangiologica Europa* **53** (6), pp. 537–547.

Menash G A, Mokdad A H, Ford E S, Greenlund K J and Croft J B (2005) State of disparities in cardiovascular health in the United States. *Circulation* **111** (10), pp. 1233–1241.

Meredith P A and Östergren J (2006) From hypertension to heart failure – Are there better primary prevention strategies? *Journal of the Renin-Angiotensin-Aldosterone System* **7** (2), pp. 64–73.

MERIT-HF Study Group (1999) Effect of metoprolol CR/XL in chronic heart failure: metoprolol CR/XL randomised intervention trial in congestive heart failure (MERIT-HF). *The Lancet* **353** (9169), pp. 2001–2007.

Merritt S L (2004) Sleep disordered breathing and the association with cardiovascular risk. *Progress in Cardiovascular Nursing* **19** (1), pp. 19–27.

Meyer J A (1990) Werner Forssmann and catheterization of the heart, 1929. *The Annals of Thoracic Surgery* **49** (3), pp. 497–499.

Meyer F J, Borst M M, Zugck C, Kirscke A, Schellberg D, Kubler W and Haass M (2001) Respiratory muscle dysfunction in congestive heart failure: clinical correlation and prognostic significance. *Circulation* **103** (17), pp. 2153–2158.

Meyer T E, Casadei B, Coats A J S, Davey P P, Adamopoulos S, Radaelli A et al. (1991) Angiotensin converting enzyme inhibition and physical training in heart failure. *Journal of Internal Medicine* **230** (5), pp. 407–413.

Michalson A, Konig G and Thimme W (1998) Preventable causative factors leading to hospital admission with decompensated heart failure. *Heart* **80** (5), pp. 437–441.

Middlekauff H R, Stevenson W G and Saxon L A (1993) Prognosis after syncope: impact of left ventricular function. *American Heart Journal* **125** (1), pp. 121–127.

Mølgaard H, Kristensen B O and Baandrup U (1990) Importance of abstention from alcohol in alcoholic heart disease. *International Journal of Cardiology* **26** (3), pp. 373–375.

Morrison, D (2006) PCI versus CABG versus medical therapy in 2006. *Minerva Cardioangiologica Europa* **54** (5), pp. 643–672.

Moser D K, Lennie T A and Doering L V (2004) Non-pharmacologic management of heart failure. In Stewart S, Moser D K and Thompson D R, *Caring for the Heart Failure Patient: A Textbook for the Health Care Professional.* London: Martin Dunitz.

Moser D K, Doering L V and Chung M L (2005) Vulnerabilities of patients recovering from an exacerbation of chronic heart failure. *American Heart Journal* **150** (5), p. 984.

Moss A J, Zareba W, Jackson Hall W, Klein H, Wilber D J, Cannon D S et al. (2002) Prophylactic implantation of a defibrillator in patients with myocardial infarction and reduced ejection fraction. *The New England Journal of Medicine* **346** (12), pp. 877–883.

Mosterd A, Hoes A W, deBruyne M C, Deckers J W, Linker J W, Hofman A and Grobbee D E (1999) Prevalence of heart failure and left ventricular dysfunction in the general population: the Rotterdam Study. *European Heart Journal* **20** (6), pp. 447–455.

Mukamal K J, Tolstrup J S, Friberg J, Jenson G and Grønbaek M (2005) Alcohol consumption and risk of atrial fibrillation in men and women: the Copenhagen City Heart Study. *Circulation* **112** (12), pp. 1736–1742.

Murphy R T and Starling R T (2005) Genetics and cardiomyopathy: Where are we now? *Cleveland Clinic Journal of Medicine* **72** (6), pp. 465–483.

Murray S A, Boyd K, Kendall M, Worth A, Benson T F and Clausen H (2002) Dying of lung cancer or cardiac failure: prospective qualitative interview study of patients and their carers in the community. *British Medical Journal* **325** (7370), pp. 929–932.

Nazarian S, Maisel W H, Miles J S, Tsang S, Stevenson L W and Stevenson W G (2005) Impact of implantable cardioverter defibrillators on survival and recurrent hospitalisation in advanced heart failure. *American Heart Journal* **150** (5), pp. 955–960.

Ng E, Stafford P J and Ng G A (2004) Arrhythmia detection by patient and auto-activation in implantable loop recorders. *Journal of Interventional Cardiac Electrophysiology* **10** (2), pp. 147–152.

NICE (2003) *Chronic Heart Failure: National Clinical Guideline for Diagnosis and Management in Primary and Secondary Care*, NICE: London.

Nicklas B J, Cesari M, Penninx B M J, Kritchevsky S B, Ding J, Newman A et al. (2006) Abdominal obesity is an independent risk factor for chronic heart failure in older people. *Journal of the American Geriatrics Society* **54** (3), pp. 413–420.

Nicolozakes A W, Binkley P F and Leier C V (1988) Haemodynamic effects of smoking in congestive cardiac failure. *American Journal of Medical Science* **296** (6), pp. 377–380.

North T C, McCullough P and Tran Z V (1990) Effect of exercise on depression. *Exercise Sport Science Review* **18** (1), pp. 379–415.

O'Neill T W, Barry M, Smith M and Graham I M (1989) Diagnostic value of the apex beat. *Lancet* **2** (8661), pp. 410–11.

Oshima K, Morishita Y, Hinohara H, Kadoi Y, Hayashi Y, Tajima Y and Kunimoto F (2005) Prolonged use for at least ten days of intraaortic balloon pumping (IABP) for heart failure. *International Heart Journal* **46** (6), pp. 1041–1047.

Pachori A S, Melo L G and Dzau V J (2006) Gene therapy: role in myocardial protection. *Handbook of Experimental Pharmacology* **176** (2), pp. 335–350.

Packer M, Gheorghiade M, Young J B, Costantini P J, Adams K F, Cody R J et al. (1993) Withdrawal of digoxin from patients with chronic heart failure treated with angiotensin-converting-enzyme inhibitors. RADIANCE Study. *The New England Journal of Medicine* **329** (1), pp. 1–7.

Packer M, Bristow M R, Cohn J N, Colucci W S, Fowler M B, Gilbert E M et al. (1996) The effect of carvedilol on morbidity and mortality in patients with chronic heart failure. US Carvedilol Heart Failure Study Group. *The New England Journal of Medicine* **334** (21), pp. 1349–1355.

Packer M, Poole-Wilson P A, Armstrong P W, Cleland J G, Horowitz J D, Massie B M et al. (1999) Comparative effects of low and high doses of the angiotensin-converting enzyme inhibitor, lisinopril, on morbidity and mortality in chronic heart failure. ATLAS Study Group. *Circulation* **100** (23), pp. 2312–2318.

Packer M, Abraham W T, Mehra M R, Yancy C W, Lawless C E, Mitchell J E et al. (2006) Utility of impedance cardiography for the identification of short-term risk of clinical decompensation in stable patients with chronic heart failure. *Journal of the American College of Cardiology* **47** (11), pp. 2245–2252.

Palmer N D, Appleton B and Rodrigues E A (2003) Specialist nurse-led intervention in outpatients with congestive heart failure: impact on clinical and economic outcomes. *Disease Management Health Outcomes* **11** (11), pp. 693–698.

Panina G, Khot U N, Nunziata E, Cody R J and Binkley P F (1995) Assessment of autonomic tone over a 24-hour period in patients with congestive heart failure: relation between mean heart rate and measures of heart rate variability. *American Heart Journal* **129** (4), pp. 748–753.

Parikh S and de Lemos J A (2005) Current therapeutic strategies in cardiac amyloidosis. *Current Treatment Options in Cardiovascular Medicine* **7** (6), pp. 443–448.

Park E W, Schultz J K, Tudiver F, Campbell T and Becker L (2004) Enhancing partner support to improve smoking cessation. *Cochrane Database of Systematic Reviews,* **3**.

Partridge G (2004) Echocardiography in the community: mind the gap. *British Journal of Cardiology* **11** (5), pp. 403–404.

Patel A N, Geffner L, Vina R F, Saslavsky J, Urschel H C Jnr, Kormos R and Benneti F (2005) Surgical treatment for congestive heart failure with autologous adult stem cell transplantation: a prospective randomised study. *Journal of Thoracic Cardiovascular Surgery* **130** (6), pp. 1631–1638.

Patel R, Bushness D L and Sobotka P A (1993) Implications of an audible third heart sound in evaluating cardiac function. *The Western Journal of Medicine* **158** (6), pp. 606–609.

Peacock W F, Albert N M, White R D and Emerman C L (2000) Bioimpedance monitoring: better than chest x-ray for predicting abnormal pulmonary fluid? *Congestive Heart Failure* **6** (2), pp. 86–89.

Perin E, Dohmann H F R, Borojevic R, Silva S A, Sousa A L S, Mesquita C T et al. (2003) Transendocardial, autologous bone marrow cell transplantation for severe, chronic ischaemic heart failure. *Circulation* **107** (18), pp. 2294–2302.

Persson H, Ionn E, Edner M, Barach L, Lang C C, Morton J J et al. (2007) Diastolic dysfunction in heart failure with preserved systolic function: need for objective evidence: results from the CHARM echocardiographic sub study – CHARMES. *Journal of the American College of Cardiology* **49** (6), pp. 687–694.

Pfeffer M A, Braunwald E, Moye L A, Basta L, Brown E J Jnr, Cuddy T E et al. (1992) Effect of captopril on mortality and morbidity in patients with left ventricular dysfunction after myocardial infarction. Results of the survival and ventricular enlargement trial. The SAVE investigators. *The New England Journal of Medicine* **327** (10), pp. 669–677.

Phillips C O, Singa R M, Rubin H R and Jaarsma T (2005) Complexity of program and clinical outcomes of heart failure disease management incorporating specialist nurse-led heart failure clinics. A meta-regression analysis. *European Journal of Heart Failure* **7** (3), pp. 333–341.

Piano M R (2002) Alcoholic cardiomyopathy: incidence, clinical characteristics, and pathophysiology. *Chest* **121** (5), pp. 1638–1650.

Piano M R and Schwertz D W (1994) Alcoholic heart disease: a review. *Heart and Lung* **23** (1), pp. 3–17.

Piepoli M F, Flather M and Coats A J S (1998a) Overview of studies of exercise training in chronic heart failure: the need for a prospective multicentre European trial. *European Heart Journal* **19** (6), pp. 830–841.

Piepoli M, Villani G Q, Ponikowski P, Wright A, Falther M D and Coats A J (1998b) Overview and meta-analysis of randomised trials of amiodarone in chronic heart failure. *International Journal of Cardiology* **66** (1), pp. 1–10.

Piepoli M F, Davos C, Francis D P and Coats A J S (2004) Exercise training meta-analysis of trials in patients with chronic heart failure (ExTraMATCH). *British Medical Journal* **328** (7433), pp. 189–196.

Pitt B, Segal R, Martinez F A, Meurers G, Cowley A J, Thomas I et al. (1997) Randomised trial of losartan versus captopril in patients over 65 with heart failure (Evaluation of Losartan in the Elderly study, ELITE). *The Lancet* **349** (9054), pp. 747–752.

Pitt B, White H, Nicolau J, Martinez F, Gheorghiade M, Aschermann M et al. (2005) Eplerenone reduces mortality 30 days after randomization following acute myocardial infarction in patients with left ventricular systolic dysfunction and heart failure. *Journal of the American College of Cardiology* **46** (3), pp. 425–31.

Pocar M, Moneta A, Adalberto G and Donatelli F (2007) Coronary artery bypass for heart failure in ischemic cardiomyopathy: 17-year follow-up. *The Annals of Thoracic Surgery* **83** (2), pp. 468–474.

Poole-Wilson P A, Swedberg K, Cleland J G F, DiLenarda A, Hanrath P, Komajada M et al. (2003) Comparison of carvedilol and metoprolol on clinical outcomes in patients with chronic heart failure in the carvedilol or metoprolol European trial (COMET): randomised controlled trial. *The Lancet* **362** (9377), pp. 7–13.

Powell B D, Redfield M M, Bybee K A, Freeman W K and Rihal C S (2006) Association of obesity with left ventricular remodeling and diastolic dysfunction in patients without coronary artery disease. *The American Journal of Cardiology* **98** (1), pp. 116–120.

Pu C T, Johnson M T, Forman D E, Hausdorff J M, Roubenoff R and Foldarvi M (2001) Randomised trial of progressive resistance to exercise training to counteract the myopathy of chronic heart failure. *Journal of Applied Physiology* **90** (6), pp. 2341–2350.

Ramasamy R, Hildebrandt T, O'Hea E, Patel M, Clemow L, Freudenberger R and Skotzko C (2006) Psychological and social factors that correlate with dyspnoea in heart failure. *Psychosomatics* **47** (5), pp. 430–434.

Rector T S, Anand I S and Cohn J N (2006) Relationships between clinical assessments and patients' perceptions of the effects of heart failure on their quality of life. *Journal of Cardiac Failure* **12** (2), pp. 87–92.

Remes J, Miettinen H, Reunanen A and Pyorala K (1991) Validity of clinical diagnosis of heart failure in primary health care. *European Heart Journal* **12** (3), pp. 315–321.

Rexrode, K M, Carey, V J, Hennekems, C H et al. (1998) Abdominal adiposity and coronary heart disease in women. *Journal of the American Heart Association* **280** (21), pp. 1843–1848.

Rich M W, McSherry F, Williford W O and Yusuf S (2001) Effect of age on mortality, hospitalizations and response to digoxin in patients with heart failure: the DIG study. *Journal of the American College of Cardiology* **38** (3), pp. 806–813.

Rosanio S, Schwartz E R, Ahmad M, Jammula P, Vitarelli A, Uretsky B F et al. (2005) Benefits, unresolved questions, and technical issues of cardiac resynchronization therapy for heart failure. *The American Journal of Cardiology* **96** (5), pp. 710–717.

Rose E A, Gelijns A C, Moskowitz A J, Heitjan D F, Stevenson L W Dembtsky W et al. (2001) Long term mechanical left ventricular assistance for end stage heart failure. Randomised evaluation of mechanical assistance for the treatment of congestive heart failure study. *The New England Journal of Medicine* **345** (20), pp. 1435–1443.

Rumsfeld J S, Jones P G, Whooley M A, Sullivan M D, Pitt B, Weintraub W S et al. (2005) Depression predicts mortality and hospitalisation in patients with myocardial infarction complicated by heart failure. *American Heart Journal* **150** (5), pp. 961–967.

Salisbury A C, House J A, Conrad M W, Krumholtz H M and Spertus J A (2005) Low to moderate alcohol intake and health status in heart failure patients. *Journal of Cardiac Failure* **11** (5), pp. 328–328.

Saxon L A, Bristow M R, Boehmer J, Krueger S, Kass D A De Marco T et al. (2006) Predictors of sudden cardiac death and appropriate shock in the Comparison of Medical Therapy, Pacing, and Defibrillation in Heart Failure (COMPANION) Trial. *Circulation* **114** (25), pp. 2766–2772.

Scalvini S, Zanelli E, Volterrani M, Martinelli G, Baratti D, Buscaya O, Baiardi P, Glisenti F and Giodano A (2004) A pilot study of nurse led, home based telecardiology for patients with chronic heart failure. *Journal of Telemedicine and Telecare* **10** (2), pp. 113–117.

Schellenbaum G D, Rea T D, Heckbert S R, Smith N L, Lumley T, Roger V L et al. (2004) Survival associated with two sets of diagnostic criteria for congestive heart failure. *American Journal of Epidemiology* **160** (7), pp. 628–635.

Schmitt B P, Kusher M S and Weiner S L (1986) The diagnostic usefulness of the history of the patient with dyspnoea. *Journal of General Internal Medicine* **1** (6), pp. 386–393.

Schocken D D, Arrieta M I, Leaverton P E and Ross E A (1992) Prevalence and mortality rate of congestive heart failure in the United States. *Journal of the American College of Cardiology* **20** (2), pp. 301–306.

Sekiguchi M, Yazaki Y, Isobe M and Hiroe M (1996) Cardiac sarcoidosis: diagnostic, prognostic, and therapeutic considerations. *Cardiovascular Drugs and Therapy* **10** (5), pp. 495–510.

Senni M, Tribouilloy C M, Rodeheffer R J, Jacobsen S J, Evans J M, Bailey K R et al. (1999) Congestive heart failure in the community: trends in incidence and survival in a 10 year period. *Archives of Internal Medicine* **159** (1), pp. 29–34.

Sesti C and Kloner R A (2004) Gene therapy in congestive heart failure. *Circulation* **110** (3), pp. 242–243.

Seth R, Magner P, Matzinger F and van Walraven C (2002) How far is the sternal angle from the mid right atrium? *Journal of General Internal Medicine* **17** (11), pp. 852–856.

Shah M R, Flavell C M, Weintraub J R, Young M A, Hasselblad V, Fang J C et al. (2005) Intensity and focus of heart failure disease management after hospital discharge. *American Heart Journal* **149** (4), pp. 715–721.

Sharpe N and Doughty R (1998) Epidemiology of heart failure and ventricular dysfunction. *The Lancet* **353** S1, S3–7.

Shepler S A and Patel A N (2007) Cardiac cell therapy: a treatment option for cardiomyopathy. *Critical Care Nursing Quarterly* **30** (1), pp. 74–80.

Sherwood A, Blumenthal J A, Trivedi R, Johnson K S, O'Connor C M, Adams K F Jr et al. (2007) Relationship of depression to death or hospitalization in patients with heart failure. *Archives of Internal Medicine* **167** (4), pp. 367–373.

Shin D D, Brandimarte F, DeLuca L, Sabbah H N, Fonarow G C, Filippatos G et al. (2007) Review of current and investigational pharmacologic agents for acute heart failure syndromes. *American Journal of Cardiology* **99** (2), pp. S4–23.

SIGN (2007) *Management of Chronic Heart Failure: a National Clinical Guideline*, Edinburgh: Scottish Intercollegiate Guidelines Network.

Sinoway L I (1988) Effects of conditioning and deconditioning stimuli on metabolically determined blood flow in humans and implications for congestive heart failure. *American Journal of Cardiology* **62** 45E–48E.

Sneed N V and Paul S C (2003) Readiness for behavioural changes in patients with heart failure. **1** (5), pp. 444–453.

Solomon S D, Anavekar N, Skali H, McMurray J J, Swedberg K, Yusuf S et al. (2005) Influence of ejection fraction on cardiovascular outcomes in a broad spectrum of heart failure patients. *Circulation* **112** (24), pp. 3738–3744.

Sosin M D, Bhatia G S, Davis R C and Lip G Y H (2004) Heart failure – the importance of ethnicity. *European Journal of Heart Failure* **6** (7), pp. 831–843.

Spies C D, Sander M, Stangl K, Fernandez S J, Preedy V R, Rubin E et al. (2001) Effects of alcohol on the heart. *Current Opinion in Critical Care* **7** (5), pp. 337–343.

Spyrou N and Foale R (1994) Restrictive cardiomyopathies. *Current Opinion in Cardiology* **9** (3), pp. 344–348.

Squires R W (1985) Moderate altitude exposure and the cardiac patient. *Journal of Cardiopulmonary Rehabilitation* **5** (9), pp. 421–426.

Stevenson W G and Tedrow U (2006) Management of atrial fibrillation in patients with heart failure. *Heart Rhythm* **4** (3), pp. S28–S30.

Stewart A (1989) Functional status and well being of patients with chronic conditions. *Journal of the American Medical Association* **262** (7), pp. 907–913.

Stewart S and Blue L (2001) *Improving Outcomes in Chronic Heart Failure: a practical guide to specialist nurse intervention,* London: BMJ Books.

Stewart S and Horowitz J D (2003) Specialist nurse management programmes: economic benefits in the management of heart failure. *Pharmacoeconomics* **21** (4), pp. 225–240.

Stewart S, Pearson S and Horowitz J D (1998) Effects of a home based intervention among patients with congestive heart failure discharged from acute hospital care. *Archives of Internal Medicine* **158** (10), pp. 1067–1072.

Stewart S, Vandenbroeak A J, Pearson S and Horowitz J D (1999) Prolonged beneficial effects of a home based intervention on unplanned readmissions and mortality among patients with congestive heart failure. *Archives of Internal Medicine* **159** (3), pp. 257–261.

Stewart S, MacIntyre K, Hole D J, Capewell S and McMurray J J (2001) More 'malignant' than cancer? Five-year survival following a first admission for heart failure. *European Journal of Heart Failure* **3** (3), pp. 315–322,

Stewart S, Blue L, Walker A, Morrison C and McMurray J J V (2002) An economic analysis of specialist heart failure nurse management in the UK. Can we afford not to implement it? *European Heart Journal* **23** (17), pp. 1369–1378.

Stewart S, MacIntyre K, Capewell S and McMurray J J V (2003) Heart failure and the aging population: an increasing burden in the 21st century? *Heart* **89** (1), pp. 49–53.

Stramba-Badiale M, Fox K M, Priori S G, Collins P, Daly C, Graham L et al. (2006) Cardiovascular disease in women: a statement from the policy conference of the European Society of Cardiology. *European Heart Journal* **27** (8), pp. 994–1005.

Struthers A D (2000) The diagnosis of heart failure. *Heart* **84** (3), pp. 334–338.

Subramanian U, Weiner M, Gradus P, Jingwel W and Murray M D (2005) Patient perception and provider assessment of severity of heart failure as predictors of hospitalisation. *Heart and Lung* **34** (2), pp. 89–98.

Sullivan M J, Higginbottom M B and Cobb F R (1989) Exercise training in patients with chronic heart failure delays ventricular aerobic threshold and improves submaximal exercise performance. *Circulation* **79** (2), pp. 324–329.

Summers R L, Peacock W F, Vogel J and Emerman C E (2006) Impact of impedance cardiography on diagnosis and therapy of emergent dyspnea: the ED-IMPACT trial. *Academic Emergency Medicine* **13** (4), pp. 365–371.

Suskin N, Sheth T, Negassa A and Yusuf S (2001) Relationship of current and past smoking to mortality and morbidity in patients with left ventricular dysfunction. *Journal of the American College of Cardiology* **37** (6), pp. 1677–1682.

Swedberg K, Kjekshus J and Snapinn S (1999) Long-term survival in severe heart failure in patients treated with enalapril. Ten year follow-up of CONSENSUS I. *European Heart Journal* **20** (2), pp. 136–139.

Swedberg K, Cleland J, Dargie H, Drexler H, Follath F, Komajda M et al. (2005) Guidelines for the diagnosis and treatment of chronic heart failure: executive summary. *European Heart Journal* **26** (11), pp. 1115–1140.

Tenenbaum A, Freimark D, Ahron E, Koren M N, Schwamenthal E, Fisman E Z et al. (2006) Long-term versus intermediate-term supervised exercise training in advanced heart failure: effects on exercise tolerance and mortality. *International Journal of Cardiology* **113** (3), pp. 364–370.

Teragaki M, Takeuchi K and Takeda T (1993) Clinical and histologic features of alcohol drinkers with congestive heart failure. *American Heart Journal* **125** (3), pp. 808–817.

The AIRE Study Investigators (1993) Effect of ramipril on mortality and morbidity of survivors of acute myocardial infarction with clinical evidence of heart failure. *The Lancet* **342** (8875), pp. 821–828.

The Antiarrhythmics versus Implantable Defibrillators (AVID) Investigators (1997) A comparison of antiarrythmic-drug therapy with implantable defibrillators in patients resuscitated from near-fatal ventricular arrhythmias. *The New England Journal of Medicine* **337** (22), pp. 1576–1583.

The Australia-New Zealand Heart Failure Research Collaborative Group (1995) Effects of carvedilol, a vasodilator-beta-blocker, in patients with congestive heart failure due to ischemic heart disease. *Circulation* **92** (2), pp. 212–218.

The CIBIS-II Investigators (1999) The cardiac insufficiency bisoprolol study II (CIBIS-II): a randomised trial. *The Lancet* **353** (9146), pp. 9–13.

The HOPE Study Investigators (2000) Effects of an angiotensin-converting-enzyme inhibitor, ramipril, on cardiovascular events in high-risk patients. *The New England Journal of Medicine* **342** (3), pp. 145–153.

The MERIT-HF Investigators (1999) Effects of metoprolol CR/XL in chronic heart failure: metoprolol CR/XL randomised intervention trial in congestive heart failure (MERIT-HF). *The Lancet* **353** (9169), pp. 2001–2007.

The RALES Investigators (1996) Effectiveness of spironolactone added to an angiotensin-converting enzyme inhibitor and a loop diuretic for severe chronic congestive heart failure (the Randomized Aldactone Evaluation Study (RALES)). *The American Journal of Cardiology* **78** (8), pp. 902–7.

The SOLVD Investigators (1991) Effect of enalapril on survival in patients with reduced left ventricular ejection fractions and congestive heart failure. *The New England Journal of Medicine* **325** (5), pp. 293–302.

The SUPPORT Principal Investigators (1995) A controlled trial to improve care for seriously ill hospitalized patients. The study to understand prognoses and preferences for outcomes and risks of treatments (SUPPORT). *The Journal of the American Medical Association* **274** (20), pp. 1591–1598.

The United Kingdom Prospective Diabetic Study Group (1998) Effect of intensive blood-glucose control with metformin on complications in overweight patients with type 2 diabetes (UKPDS 34). *The Lancet* **352** (9131), pp. 854–865.

Thomas K L and Velazquez E J (2005) Therapies to prevent heart failure post-myocardial infarction. *Current Heart Failure Reports* **2** (4), pp. 174–182.

Thompson D R, Bowman G S, Kitson A L, de Bono D P and Hopkins A (1997) Cardiac rehabilitation services in England and Wales: a national survey. *International Journal of Cardiology* **59** (3), pp. 299–304.

Thompson D R, Rosebuck A and Stewart S (2005) Effects of a nurse-led, clinic and home-based intervention on recurrent hospital use in chronic heart failure. *European Journal of Heart Failure* **7** (3), pp. 377–384.

Uretsky B F, Young J B, Shahidi F E, Yellen L G, Harrison M C and Jolly M K (1993) Randomized study assessing the effect of digoxin withdrawal in patients with mild to moderate chronic congestive heart failure: results of the PROVED trial. PROVED Investigative Group. *Journal of the American College of Cardiology* **22** (4), pp. 955–962.

UK Transplant (2007) http://www.uktransplant.org.uk/ukt/statistics/statistics.jsp

Van Jaarsveld C H M, Ranchor A V, Kempen G I J M, Coyne J C, Van Veldhuisem D J and Sanderman R (2006) Epidemiology of heart failure in a community-based study of subjects aged > or = 57 years: incidence and long-term survival. *European Journal of Heart Failure* **8** (1), pp. 23–30.

Veinot J P and Johnston B (1998) Cardiac sarcoidosis – an occult cause of sudden death: a case report and literature review. *Journal of Forensic Sciences* **43** (3), pp. 715–717.

Ventura H O and Mehra M R (2005) Bloodletting as a cure for dropsy: heart failure down the ages. *Journal of Cardiac Failure* **11** (4), pp. 247–252.

Visser L and Purday J (1998) Management of cardiogenic shock in a district general hospital. *Care of the Critically Ill* **14** (7), pp. 240–244.

Volpe M, Tritto C and DeLuca N (1993) Abnormalities of sodium handling and of cardiovascular adaptations during high salt intake in patients with mild heart failure. *Circulation* **88** (4 part 1), pp. 1620–1627.

Waagstein F, Bristow M R, Swedberg K, Camerini F, Fowler M B, Silver M A, et al. (1993) Beneficial effects of metoprolol in idiopathic dilated cardiomyopathy. Metoprolol in Dilated Cardiomyopathy (MDC) Trial Study Group. *The Lancet* **342** (8885), pp. 1441–1446.

Walsh C R and Levy D (2003) Alcohol and congestive cardiac failure. Letter. *Annals of Internal Medicine* **138** (1), pp. 75–6.

Wang R Y, Alterman A I, Searless J S and MacLellan A T (1990) Alcohol abuse in patients with dilated cardiomyopathy. *Archives of Internal Medicine* **150** (5), pp. 1079–1082.

Watson R D S, Gibbs C R and Lipp G Y A (2000) ABC of heart failure: clinical features and complications. *British Medical Journal* **320** (7229), pp. 236–239.

Widimsky P, Penicka M, Lang O, Kozak T, Motovska Z, Jirmar R and Aschermann M (2006) Intracoronary transplantation of bone marrow stem cells: background, techniques, and limitations. *European Heart Journal* **8** Supplement, H16–22.

Williams B, Poulter N R, Brown M J, Davis M, McInnes G T, Potter J P et al. (2004) The BHS Guidelines Working Party Guidelines for Management of Hypertension: Report of the Fourth Working Party of the British Hypertension Society. *Journal of Human Hypertension* **18** (3), pp. 139–185.

Williams N (2003) Nurse led transitional care improved health related quality of life and reduced emergency department use for heart failure. *Evidence-Based Nursing* **6** (1), p. 21.

Winkens, R and Dinant, G-J (2002) Rational, cost effective use of investigations in clinical practice. *British Medical Journal* **324** (7340), pp. 783–785.

Witham M D, Gillespie N D and Struthers A D (2004) Age is not a significant risk factor for failed trial of beta-blocker therapy in older patients with chronic heart failure. *Age and Aging* **33** (5), pp. 467–472.

Wolk R, Gami A S, Garcia-Touchard A and Somers V K (2005) Sleep and cardiovascular disease. *Current Problems in Cardiology* **30** (12), pp. 625–662.

Wong B and Rattery M P (2006) Use of digoxin in the treatment of chronic heart failure. *Progress in Cardiovascular Nursing* **21** (3), pp. 158–161.

World Health Organization (1980) Report of the WHO/ISFC Task Force on the Definitions and Classifications of Cardiomyopathies. *British Heart Journal* **44** (6), pp. 672–673.

Yao G, Freemantle N, Calvert M J, Stirling B, Daubert J C and Cleland J G F (2007) The long-term cost-effectiveness of cardiac resynchronization therapy with or without an implantable cardioverter-defibrillator. *European Heart Journal* **28** (1), pp. 42–51.

Young J B, Abraham W T, Smith A L, Leon A R, Liberman R, Wilkoff B et al. (2003) Combined cardiac resynchronization and implantable cardioversion defibrillation in advanced chronic heart failure: the MIRACLE ICD Trial. *The Journal of the American Medical Association* **289** (20), pp. 2685–2694.

Ypenburg C, Bax J J, van der Wall E E, Schalij M J and van Eryen I (2007) Intrathoracic impedance monitoring to predict decompensated heart failure. *American Journal of Cardiology* **99** (4), pp. 554–557.

Yu D S, Thompson D R and Lee D T (2005) Disease management programmes for older people with heart failure: crucial characteristics which improve post discharge outcomes. *European Heart Journal* **27** (9), pp. 596–612.

Yusuf S, Pfeffer M A, Swedberg K, Granger C B, Held P, McMurray J J V et al (2003) Effects of candesartan in patients with chronic heart failure and preserved left ventricular ejection fraction: the CHARM-Preserved Trial. *The Lancet* **362** (9386), pp. 777–781.

Zannad F, Briancon S, Juilliere Y, Mertes P-M, Villemot J-P, Alla F, et al. (1999) Incidence, clinical and etiologic features, and outcomes of advanced heart failure: the EPICAL study. *Journal of the American College of Cardiology* **33** (3), pp. 734–42.

Index